TINNITUS:
A Guide for Sufferers and Professionals

WHEN SILENCE IS SILVER . . .

For life, I am to go around
To the high-pitched sound
of a constant drill;
whizzing, whirring, never still,
until at night,
when in my bed,
I feel it boring through my head!

Seeming louder,
screaming, whining,
till I see it,
SILVER, SHINING,
Mark the thickness
of its thread . . .

Once I loved the silence so,
yet never-more such bliss shall know.
"WHAT IS THIS SUBTLE TORTURE
FOR WHICH THERE IS NO CURE?"
        "— TINNITUS!"

Years have passed . . .
Sweet hope at last
appears for such as I!
As members of the BTA.,
we dare to question fixed belief;
"WHY SHOULD WE LIVE WITHOUT RELIEF
UNTIL THE DAY WE DIE?"

If all the noises we endure
were sounding out externally,
there could not then be apathy.
Even hardened souls in HELL
would all cry out alarmingly
for
        "MERCY! Or a cure!"

                                        Joan Neininger 1981

(sent in with a completed tinnitus research questionnaire)

TINNITUS:

A Guide for Sufferers and Professionals

ROBERT SLATER AND MARK TERRY
With a chapter by BRIAN DAVIS

CROOM HELM
London & Sydney

© 1987 Robert Slater and Mark Terry
Croom Helm Ltd, Provident House, Burrell Row,
Beckenham, Kent BR3 1AT

Croom Helm Australia, 44–50 Waterloo Road,
North Ryde, 2113, New South Wales

British Library Cataloguing in Publication Data

Slater, Robert
    Tinnitus: a guide for sufferers and professionals
    1. Tinnitus
    I. Title   II. Terry, Mark
    617.8   RF293.8
    ISBN 0–7099–3338–X
    ISBN 0–7099–3339–8 Pbk

Distributed exclusively in the USA by Sheridan House Inc.,
145 Palisade Street, Dobbs Ferry NY 10522

Filmset by Mayhew Typesetting, Bristol, England
Printed and bound in Great Britain by Mackays of Chatham Ltd, Kent

Dedication

This book is dedicated to Mary, Tom and Frank, who, among many other far worse things, had to put up with a table-tennis table covered in manuscripts and papers for the two years this book was in preparation.

Contents

ABOUT THE AUTHORS

Robert Slater is a lecturer in Psychology at UWIST, Cardiff. He obtained a B.A. in Developmental Psychology in 1966 and an M.Phil. in Social Psychology in 1968, both from Sussex University. After a short spell at the University of Liverpool and Manchester Polytechnic he 'settled down' at UWIST in 1970. Most of his research has involved the evaluation of service provisions for disadvantaged individuals — often those for older people. His research interest in tinnitus developed after he himself became a 'sufferer' in 1975. He has been chairman of his local tinnitus self-help group for the past five years and he is involved in counselling people with tinnitus. He is married to a health authority administrator, Mary, and has two sons, Tom 7 and Frank 3, and another one on the way.

Brian Davis is a Consultant E.N.T. Surgeon practising in West Wales. He qualified in medicine at the Westminster Hospital, London in 1972 and obtained the Fellowship of the Royal College of Surgeons of England in 1978. After working in London and Bristol he completed his higher specialist training at the University Hospital of Wales in Cardiff. It was whilst at Cardiff that he developed a particular interest in tinnitus and became a member of the research team at UWIST, upon whose findings much of this book is based.

Mark Terry was a postdoctoral research worker on our DHSS-funded study. He obtained a PhD in psychology from Reading University in 1981 and is currently Research Fellow at the Centre for Speech Technology Research, University of Edinburgh.

Figures

Tables

Preface

Almost everyone has experienced a short, faint, ringing in the ears at some time or other. For some the noise would come and go 'out of the blue', others may have noticed it after listening to loud music or after any really loud sudden noise. Some people have such noises in their ear or ears, or seemingly inside their head, *all* the time, and the noise or noises may have started apparently 'out of the blue' too. Some people have noises that are far from faint but sound very loud indeed to them. All such noises are referred to as 'tinnitus' or 'head noises'. In a large proportion of individuals these noises cannot be heard by others even with the use of the most sophisticated equipment. Somehow, in people with tinnitus, the mechanisms in the ear and the brain that are part of our hearing processes are able to generate the electrical signals that normally are a response to noise that *is* there, even when external noise isn't there. In a way this is rather like many record players that will generate some noise if turned up to a very high volume, even when a record isn't being played, although this analogy cannot be taken very far. Individuals' reactions to continuous, loud, piercing forms of tinnitus are usually, and understandably, negative; anxiety and depression often follow, particularly when it appears that the tinnitus will remain with the individual for the rest of his or her life and it is suggested that little can be done to help.

This book aims to present what is currently known about tinnitus, its causes and effects, and ways that *are* available of dealing with these, in a way that is understandable to the person who has tinnitus and his or her friends and relatives, as well as in a way that is informative to those professionals who in the course of their work will need to *respond* to individuals with tinnitus. Many 'sufferers' and specialists alike have only a sketchy appreciation of the complexities of the condition, and certainly for the sufferer ignorance is far from bliss — it leads only to increased worry and stress and to a feeling of impotence in the professional who does want to be able to help. We hope this book will help both.

Acknowledgements

This book derives some of its data from a (DHSS-funded) research project carried out by the authors and by Dr Dylan Jones of the Applied Psychology Department, UWIST, to whom we are grateful. Special thanks go to Viv Williams, who administered the survey side of the project as well as liaising with subjects for experiments. Thanks must also go to the 30 or so subjects who took part in our experiments and the 984 people who completed our research questionnaire. Liz and Debbie made a wonderful job of the typing, coping with wholesale redrafts and tiny changes with great patience.

1

Introduction

Coping with tinnitus, for those for whom the nature of the tinnitus presents a problem, is, to a great extent, a psychological matter. Some might say in this context that a little knowledge is a dangerous thing — that tinnitus 'sufferers' are better off in a state of ignorance about the complaint because otherwise they will spend their time and efforts either worrying even more about it or chasing perhaps expensive remedies that are only too likely to be unsuccessful. Those who might argue this way may say that 'learning to live with it', though a harsh treatment, means coming to terms with the fact that nothing *can* be done about it and that the less attention there is paid to it the better — 'out of sight out of mind'. Of course most people *do* learn to live with tinnitus, but how long does it take and at what cost to the quality of their life? Could this time and cost have been lessened by them being more rather than less informed about the nature of their complaint? We believe so.

But those who feel that by providing information one may be encouraging a tendency in people to become even more preoccupied with the tinnitus do have a point. Some hearing specialists, for example, are antipathetic to self-help tinnitus groups because they believe they may ultimately cause individuals to dwell upon their problems (and those of others) more than they did before. This inherently exposes what seems at first glance to be a sort of Catch-22 element in the nature of tinnitus: you might make the problem worse by attempting to take steps to make it better.

A letter from one potential respondent to our survey questionnaire perhaps highlights this dilemma concerning tinnitus, namely that doing something about it might actually exacerbate it. The respondent wrote:

Dear Madam,

I much regret having to change my offer of cooperation in your project. I find I can only support this affliction by keeping it in the background of my thoughts. On seeing your long and detailed questionnaire I realise that I would have to accord my condition a very prominent place in my mind, and I am very reluctant to do this. To rush through and answer carelessly would be doing you no service, so I must refrain, after all, from taking part.

With apologies,

Yours sincerely,

(name supplied)

It is possible that this letter reflects the view of other people with tinnitus, who, having contacted us to say they were willing to fill out one of our research questionnaires, did not, in the event, complete the one they had been sent. Just over 1200 were distributed to people with tinnitus who had expressed a willingness to complete one, and 984 were returned completed — a response rate of 82%, which is as satisfactory as may be expected in a postal survey of this kind.

It may, then, be the case that some readers with tinnitus find that reading this book focuses their attention on the tinnitus to an extent that they find sufficiently unpleasant as to make them want to go no further. For those readers we simply hope the strength of their own curiosity about what is and is not known about tinnitus might help them overcome that temptation. Many readers will be as uninformed as was the first author when his tinnitus started — not even at the time knowing that 'tinnitus' was the word for the noise that had suddenly appeared in his right ear. Many readers may think they know as much as the family doctor, who, when invited to give a doctor's-eye-view of the tinnitus patient to a local Tinnitus Association self-help group, replied that all he knew about tinnitus could be written down on his thumb nail! Although this could not have been quite true, his reluctance to talk reflected the discontent he felt at not being able to do what doctors are supposed to do — make the patient better. It is probably such feelings of impotence that have, as Donaldson (1981) suggests, in the past made tinnitus the *bête noire* not only of those who study the ear and the nervous system, but also of psychiatrists.

SEARCHING FOR A SOLUTION

People whose tinnitus has just started often invest much energy in searching for something to get rid of it. The first author, apart from seeing his family doctor, a National Health Service ENT specialist and a private ENT specialist, insisted on seeing a psychiatrist and a consultant neurologist. With no solution coming from those medically respectable quarters he turned to other available techniques (acupuncture and hypnosis) in desperation and hope, but not on the basis of sound scientific evidence that they would be effective.

Having one's hopes raised and then dashed is perhaps worse than having no hopes at all. If that sounds unduly pessimistic let it be said now that there *are* a variety of treatments for a variety of forms of tinnitus that *are* more or less effective in helping individuals cope with the problem. But it seems clear that no magic pill to cure all tinnitus sufferers is likely to pop up in the next few years (and why this is the case will be explained later on in this book). This book is not intended to raise false aspirations but rather, by making more information readily available, it aims to help the person with tinnitus and those related to him or her, or those with a professional involvement, to understand what coping or treatment strategies *are* available, and which might work for whom and under what circumstances.

It is often said that those who haven't got tinnitus will never understand the problem it can be for those who *do* have it. Nevertheless, some specialists who have to advise people with tinnitus do appreciate its negative potential. For example Vernon (1979, p.iv) remarks that:

It's my opinion that in all the bad things that can happen to people, tinnitus is the third worst . . . The most severe and worst thing that can happen . . . is severe and intractable pain . . . The second worst is severe and intractable vertigo . . . And the third worst is severe and intractable tinnitus, for nothing robs man of the quality of life in the manner which tinnitus does . . .

And Miller (1981) states that 30 years of experience with the hearing impaired has convinced him that tinnitus causes as much suffering and anguish, if not more, than hearing loss itself. Perhaps it is Hazell (1979a, p. 470) who best describes tinnitus *in extremis*:

Many sufferers experience multiple noises apparently spread

through the head. These may change in pitch and intensity and may equal in volume the loudest sounds in our environment. It is not surprising that the most stalwart citizen may disintegrate after years of such diabolical torture and indeed suicides do occur. What is perhaps more surprising is how many sufferers manage to adapt and adjust to their tinnitus.

THE EXPERIENCE OF TINNITUS

This book will try to temper the impersonal nature of 'research results' with qualitative material that gives a perhaps better understanding of the *experience* of having tinnitus. One way, of course, of getting 'non-tinnitus persons' to experience something vaguely akin to tinnitus is to record the after-hours television sound signal or the airway noise between radio stations on a cassette tape for a continuous period of say an hour, and then play this back over light-weight headphones attached to a personal cassette player. Persons wanting the experience can then attempt to carry on whatever they were doing — to a tinnitus-like accompaniment! Perhaps the following letters, which arrived with completed tinnitus questionnaires, convey something of the personal experiences that can be associated with tinnitus:

Dear Sir,
This letter is an effort to try to give you a picture of who I am and what work I have been employed in. I am now retired and aged 65 years 5 months.

I retired in March 1980 and was employed for 39 years as a Millwright (maintenance fitter) in the foundry division of a local aircraft manufacturer. I did repairs to all kinds of moulding machines, pneumatic hammers, compressors, drop stamp hammers, forging hammers, furnaces, knock out grids, so you can deduce from that it was a very noisy place to work, most time having to shout to speak to someone.

For two years before retiring I used to say to my family that I was unable to hear my wrist watch tick with my left ear, but that did not worry me too much. Then about the end of November beginning of December 1980 I started to have a noise in my left ear, it was like the sound of air escaping from a bicycle inner tube and a whistle with it. I tolerated this through December, then in January of 1981 I decided to go to my doctor, thinking the noise was caused by wax. He examined my ear and straight away said 'You have got tinnitus and its yours for keeps', but he said 'I will send you to a specialist for a second opinion'. After waiting for weeks for an appointment I went to the nearest hospital with an ear, nose and throat department, the date, 30 March 1981. While I was there I had tests in a soundproof room, then I was taken to another place where the specialist was. He looked into my ear and confirmed it was tinnitus, then wrote a prescription for 250 Stugeron tablets, and told me to take all of them and to come back to see him on 22 May 1981. All this I faithfully did. Then I went back to hospital, the specialist asked me if the tablets had done any good, I told him no, that there was no improvement whatsoever. He expressed his regret that that was all he could do for me, then he told a nurse to make a pattern or a mould of my ear canal, and to collect it in a week's time, then to go with it to another hospital with an audio clinic. When I was there the person in attendance fitted me with a hearing aid, and after making several adjustments to it with no good results, she said 'you don't need a hearing aid', I replied 'I know, I have never asked for one'. All in all it was a complete waste of time — while I suffered this noise in my ear for months.

I was now getting depressed, and had a feeling of wanting to knock my head against a wall, however a friend of mine suggested that I try acupuncture.

This I did, so after having treatment for four to five hours once a week for three weeks the tinnitus noise has been much reduced and now I can almost forget it, sometimes the noise has gone for hours in the day. The treatment up to now has cost me £28, but it's really, for me anyway, been great.

I hope one day your team of researchers will come up with a cure, so good health to you, if there is anything I can do to help please ask.

Yours sincerely,
(name supplied)

Dear Sir or Madam,
This morning I received a cutting from the 'Guardian' (no date on it unfortunately but of course you will know what I am on about) from a friend in London a journalist (freelance) who has always been interested in me, as a sufferer — and suffer is the operative word — of that terrible condition 'tinnitus'. I have suffered from this for about 7 years. I am in my seventies and

retired in 1976 — I worked as a secretary in a Child Guidance Clinic for about 30 years and when I retired I started studying at the Open University from which I have just graduated. I am still continuing as it is my life-line — *literally* — because if I didn't study and occupy my mind, which is the only way I can to a certain extent eliminate the noises, I would and I am not dramatising this in any way, be a nervous wreck.

When I first contracted this most distressing condition about seven years ago, I woke up in the middle of the night and heard a rushing noise and thought it was cars in the road — I went to the window and there was not a car in sight. I was bewildered and terribly upset — stuffed cotton wool in my ears and finally fell asleep and woke to a normal morning — 'what a terrible nightmare I had last night' I thought. Incidentally, I am very hard of hearing — I forgot to mention this at the beginning of the letter. I went to work and then the next night it started all over again — and I have never been free from the dreadful noises since (as I write there is a loud humming going on in my ears (head?)). Yesterday, the noise was so loud — this time it was a very loud high-pitched continuous noise — in fact, I was reduced to going out of the house for a long walk — I used to have quiet days but now they grow less and less.

In the British Tinnitus Association Newsletter are many letters from tinnitus sufferers — some have confessed to desperation and suicidal feelings. I have passed that stage (I hope) but information for your Research Group I am sure can be obtained from the Newsletter. One mentioned hearing a clear tenor voice singing an aria and I have also had this experience. The woman in question called it her 'street singer' as it seemed to come from the street. Another woman told me she heard orchestras! and was desperately disturbed. I hope you don't mind my going on about the various ways in which tinnitus manifests itself. I am most curious, in spite of my sufferings, as to really what goes on — what causes the condition and when, if ever, a cure will be found — some time — never?

If I can be of any help to you, please let me know.

Yours faithfully,

(name supplied)

MANAGING TINNITUS

People who *do* 'suffer' with tinnitus may be doing themselves a disservice by considering themselves to be 'tinnitus sufferers'. Becoming a 'tinnitus sufferer' is letting tinnitus take more of a central position in one's identity than may be wise. What is more important than the sympathy that the word 'sufferer' may generate in those without tinnitus, or the self-concern and self-absorption it might generate in the person with tinnitus, is an understanding of what might exacerbate it and what might alleviate it — and why. Then one can move slowly forward from being in a passive state — from *being* a tinnitus sufferer — to an active state as the *manager* of a condition. Hazell (1979b) refers to Goodhill's earlier comment that the treatment of tinnitus as a disease is an illogical dream, but the *management* of the patient with tinnitus is an everyday necessity. This does not imply becoming obsessed with the condition and its cure, but rather becoming aware of potential strategies that might prove useful in coping with it.

Far from suggesting that the person with tinnitus has to become his own doctor, we consider that he or she has to become an active agent in changing (a) his or her own behaviour (or that of friends, relatives — and, where necessary, professionals), and (b) his or her circumstances or 'way of life', so that the deleterious effects of tinnitus on the quality of life are minimised; and this should be attempted without adopting strategies that deprive pleasures from other sources. Thus we are aiming to help individuals with tinnitus become satisfactory self-managers of their situation — using what resources are available to them. Such resources have in the past been scarce, simply because relatively little was known about tinnitus, and what *was* known was not produced for general public consumption. It is hoped that this book will be used as a resource which will go some way to rectify that situation.

THE SURVEY

Some of the information to be presented in this book arises from a survey into tinnitus undertaken on a DHSS research grant (J/S240/80/4) and appears here for the first time. Much is also taken from four technical books on tinnitus and from many journal articles. Tinnitus remains such a compact and self-contained subject area within medicine that it is relatively easy to undertake a computer-search of medical information on the subject. Such a search revealed some 400 references to articles published in the last ten years, but the majority of these were published in the last three years. This is a good sign in that it reflects the increasing interest being taken in tinnitus in both medical and audiological fields. However, much that has been written about tinnitus is based on small numbers of individuals and hence many of the findings remain inherently speculative when it comes to attempting to make generalisations. The tinnitus questionnaire survey that we undertook is no exception to this stricture.

About 40 per cent of our respondents (of the 984) were members of the British Tinnitus Association. It may well be the case that you do not readily find out about the Association's existence unless you have got as far as your family doctor or the out-patient department of your local hospital. This implies that your tinnitus may be sufficiently troublesome or worrying for you want to find out more about it. Having heard of the Tinnitus Association you may decide to join it (which requires some — albeit a minimum — effort). You then have to have sufficient interest to read its Newsletter and notice that research is being undertaken and that members are being requested to write in for a questionnaire to complete. This in itself takes an extra amount of interest, effort and dedication, and suggests a motivation to try and help do something about the situation. It is possible that those most willing to help to try and do something about it are those who find the problem most disconcerting and in this respect our sample of respondents may be biased.

The same argument applies, but perhaps to a less degree, to the 50 per cent (of our 984 respondents) who had seen a similar request in the women's page of the *Guardian* newspaper. One might argue that more women *Guardian* readers than men will read the Women's Page and that since the *Guardian* is generally considered to be a 'quality' newspaper, this group of respondents might be more middle class in composition than people in general with tinnitus.[1]

A more detailed breakdown of the sources for respondents to the questionnaire is given in Table 1.1. Suffice it to say here that any results from our survey, though interesting and suggestive in themselves, cannot be taken as statements that are necessarily true for individuals with tinnitus as a whole. In this respect some other surveys concerning tinnitus, although providing less-detailed information, can be considered to provide more generalisable results than ours (we shall detail some of their findings in Chapter 2 and elsewhere in this book). In general terms women were over-

Table 1.1: Sources of respondents to the tinnitus survey research questionnaire

Source	Number of respondents	%
British Tinnitus Association Newsletter 11	242	24.6
Local British Tinnitus Association Groups	149	15.1
Responded to a letter in the *Guardian*	514	52.9
Responded to a notice in a Suffolk newspaper	33	3.4
Friends of other respondents	6	0.6
Through an Irish hospital contact	6	0.6
Through our Medical Collaborator's list of patients	22	2.2
Untraceable	12	1.2
Total	984	100.0

Table 1.2: Main occupation of respondents

Occupation	Number of respondents	%
Professional	95	9.7
Intermediate	288	19.3
Skilled — Non-manual	200	20.3
Skilled — Manual	81	8.2
Partly skilled	47	4.8
Unskilled	11	1.1
Students	8	0.8
Retired	4	0.4
Housewife/mother	196	19.9
Unemployed	2	0.2
Otherwise unclassifiable	52	5.3
Total	984	100.0

Note: a. These groupings are from the Office of Population Censuses and Surveys' Classification of Occupations, 1980.
b. All retired people were classified according to the job they held before they retired, where this was possible.
c. Housewives with part-time jobs were classified according to their job if this seemed appropriate.

represented in our survey sample: 62 per cent of our respondents were female, 38 per cent male. A classification of respondents' jobs into broad occupational groups revealed that 10 per cent were in professional work whereas only 15 per cent were manual workers. Some could not be placed into an occupational group class on the basis of the information given in the questionnaire, and the majority of these, 19 per cent, appeared to be housewives and/or mothers.

9

Table 1.3: Age of respondents in broad age bands

Age	Number of respondents	%
39 years or younger	92	9.3
40–49 years	104	10.6
50–59 years	258	26.2
60–69 years	362	36.8
70 years or older	164	19.7
Unknown	4	0.4
Total	984	100.0

Table 1.2 gives a more detailed occupational analysis of the survey respondents.

The average age of respondents was 58 years and half the sample was aged 60 or younger. Table 1.3 gives a more detailed analysis of ages.

THE INVISIBILITY OF THE PROBLEM

Until relatively recently there has been little public awareness of tinnitus largely because of the invisibility of tinnitus as a problem. Although in some cases in terms of the suffering caused it might be analogous to incessant and prolonged pain, it does not have the outwardly observable physical consequences of pain — someone shouting out when it is particularly intense, or when they try to do something actually too painful to do. Pain brings with it many instances of physical incapacity that are observable by others. Nor is tinnitus like blindness — there is no equivalent of a white stick. Tinnitus still lags behind deafness in terms of public awareness. For the hearing-impaired there is a variety of publicly observable schemes to help: sub-titles on certain television programmes (on even more for viewers with teletext sets); schemes in shops where an ear-motif sign on entrance-doors indicates that personnel are available to give particular assistance to the hearing-impaired; the fact that people wear hearing aids (although the behind-the-ear models are designed for maximum invisibility). Often hearing-impaired people complain that *they* get little public sympathy — that 'they think if you're deaf you're daft' — yet people who hear normally *can* imagine in a crude way what it must be like to be deaf, even if they choose not to bother. In this respect tinnitus has been invisible because the condition has been almost impossible to imagine for those without it.

In previous years it is also likely that individuals with tinnitus would be unaware of just how common the problem was — since having it would not be something one would normally shout about. One reason for reticence in making public the fact that you have tinnitus are the associations and inferences others might carelessly (or out of ignorance) make. 'Hears noises or sounds in her head' can easily become 'hears voices' — and even without that twist the notion of 'hearing noises that aren't there' is uncomfortably close to some individuals' notions of the symptoms of insanity — if she hears noises she must be a bit funny-peculiar! This 'conspiracy of silence' must have led many people to feel that they were alone in having the problem, that no-one else could understand what it was like — and suffering alone was the outcome.

Also in previous years lack of public awareness has been matched by lack of noticeable interest in the topic among medical practitioners, and one reason for this might have been that, having told patients there was nothing that could be done about it, patients would go away and suffer in silence, and the doctor would remain unaware of the degree of suffering that might be being caused. We noted earlier that tinnitus has been regarded, among other things, as a *bête noire* among relevant professionals. The situation may have changed in the last few years, for both professionals and the public, because one treatment modality — maskers — has come to the fore as being potentially useful, or so it is claimed, to significant numbers of people with tinnitus, and also because organisations have set themselves up to promote awareness of the problem among professionals, public, and 'sufferers' alike.

TINNITUS ASSOCIATIONS

The British Tinnitus Association (BTA) held an inaugural meeting on 9 July 1979 at the House of Commons in London. Over 300 people attended, including an ex-Minister for the Disabled, the medical experts Jonathan Hazell from London and Jack Vernon from Portland, Oregon, as well as the British Member of Parliament, Jack Ashley, who suffered sudden deafness and associated tinnitus in middle age. By June 1984, just under five years after the BTA's inaugural meeting, membership stood at around 7000 with some 80 local self-help groups in operation. The British Tinnitus

11

Association, housed in the premises of the Royal National Institute for the Deaf (RNID), 105 Gower Street, London, publishes its own 'BTA Newsletter' (numbers 1 to 24 — September 1979 to April 1984 — being separate publications). From issue no. 25 onwards it became part of a new free quarterly RNID publication 'Sound-barrier'. The association promotes and fosters public (and professional) knowledge and interest in tinnitus as well as raising money to support further research into it.

The American Tinnitus Association (ATA), which was set up entirely by voluntary effort, is accommodated in the Kresge Hearing Research Laboratory at P.O. Box 5, Portland, Oregon 97207. In 1980 it published the ATA Newsletter, which is sent out to 14,000 tinnitus sufferers in the United States and around the world. In 1983, the ATA followed the British model of encouraging the setting up of local self-help groups. The first convention of these was held in New Jersey in June 1983, with a good many delegates attending from the over 80 recently formed local groups. The meeting agreed to the regular publication of their house journal 'The Tinnitus Trumpeter'.

Tinnitus groups also exist in the Republic of Ireland and in New Zealand, and with the success of the BTA and the ATA it is hopeful that similar associations will be set up elsewhere.

NOTES

1. Indeed, the latter proved to be true: whereas 53 per cent of the entire sample of respondents was associated with professional or 'intermediate' (semi-professional) occupations, 65 per cent of the *Guardian* respondents were so classified and this is a statistically significant difference ($\chi_2 = 55.9$, $df = 2$, P < 0.001). Surprisingly there were significantly more men than expected among *Guardian* respondents: in the overall sample 38 per cent were men, whereas 43 per cent of *Guardian* respondents were men ($\chi_2 = 12.1$, $df = 1$, P = 0.0005). Note: In several places in the text remarks will be made about a 'statistically significant difference'. These refer to the outcome of various statistical tests designed to examine how likely any differences are due purely to chance factors. Commonly the likelihood of a result being 'due to chance' — rather than to anything more tangible — is expressed as P (probability) = 0.01, for example, indicating that you could expect to get such a result by chance 1 in 100 occasions — i.e. it is not very likely to be due to chance. P = 0.001 would indicate a result occurring by chance 1 in 1000 times. The smaller the P value the less likely the result is due to chance and the more likely there is another explanation for it.

2

Sound and the ear

The ear is a marvellously complex and sensitive organ. Unfortunately, damage to that organ, whether through disease, physical insult, long term exposure to excessive noise or simply the effects of ageing, can cause the ear to malfunction. The result of the malfunction is usually to produce some degree of deafness but it may also produce tinnitus — the sensation of sound when no corresponding external sound is present. In order to understand how tinnitus arises and the way it can be best described and measured, it is helpful to gain first a basic understanding of the nature of sound and how the ear works. This is the purpose of this chapter.

It is not necessary to obtain a full understanding of all the details in this chapter before reading the rest of this book, but rather the material in the chapter should be read through once to become familiar with the contents and thereafter used for reference when required. Readers who wish a more detailed introduction to the nature of sound and the workings of the ear are referred to the bibliography section of this book.

THE NATURE OF SOUND

Sound waves

Sound is a disturbance that travels in the form of a wave through a physical medium. If a pebble is thrown into the water of a still pond a series of concentric ripples spreads out from the entry point of the pebble. The disturbance caused by the pebble travels across the surface of the pond in the form of a wave. The medium in which the wave travels is in this case water, and it is important to realise that the individual water molecules only move up and down, like a cork, and do not move across the surface (i.e. it is the disturbance that travels, not the particles of the medium). Sound also travels in the form of waves and although the usual medium is air, sound will pass through other physical materials. In fact, the denser the medium the faster the sound wave travels. For example, sound travels faster in water than in air. In a vacuum (of essentially zero density) sound will not travel.

Simple harmonic motion and the sine wave

One of the simplest sounds is the sound produced by a tuning fork or a whistle: this type of sound is known as a sinusoid or sine wave. The pattern of a sine wave vibration can be seen in Figure 2.1.

This form of vibration is also called simple harmonic motion. The same type of movement but at a much slower speed can be seen by observing a swinging pendulum or the oscillating movement of a coiled spring that is released. Air molecules will vibrate back and forth around a central position in this manner, if excited by a sound source that is vibrating in simple harmonic motion. In order to describe this motion three measurements — frequency, amplitude and phase — are needed. The frequency of a sinusoidal sound is measured in cycles per second and is the number of times the pattern of vibration repeats itself within one second.[1]

The wavelength of a sinusoid is related to the frequency and is equal to the speed of sound divided by the frequency. The period of a sine wave is simply the time taken to complete one cycle and is equal to the reciprocal of frequency. For example, a sine wave of a frequency of 1000 cycles per second (cps) has a period of 1/1000 seconds (0.001 sec) or 1 millisecond and a wavelength of approximately 33.4 cm.

wavelength = speed of sound/frequency
= 33,400 cm/sec in air/1000 Hz
= 33.4 cm

(the speed of sound will depend on the humidity, temperature and pressure of air so the above calculation is only an approximation)

Hertz (Hz) is more commonly used than cps and a frequency of 1000 cps is alternatively shown as 1000 Hz or 1 kHz (1 kiloHertz,

Figure 2.1: Sine wave

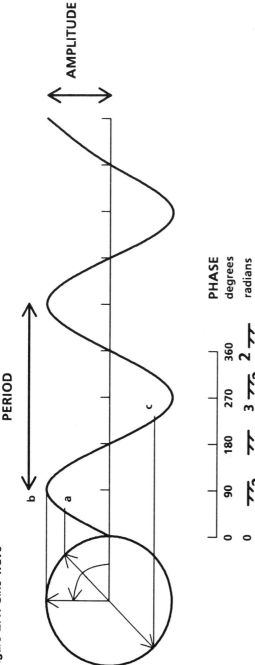

PHASE					
0	90	180	270	360	degrees
0	$\dfrac{\pi}{2}$	π	$\dfrac{3\pi}{2}$	2π	radians

The form of a sine wave and its relation to circular motion can be seen by projecting from points on the sine wave to points on the circumference of an adjacent circle (e.g. points a, b and c). If the height (amplitude) of a constantly rotating vector (like a spoke on a wheel) is plotted as a function of time, a sine wave is generated. A complete cycle is 360 degrees and the phase of the wave is shown in degrees and radians (2¼ cycles of the sine wave are shown). The period of the sine wave is the interval corresponding to one cycle (shown as the interval between two adjacent peaks in amplitude). The amplitude of the sine wave is given by $a = A \times \sin (2 \times \pi \times f \times t)$, where t = time and f = the frequency in cycles per second, A = the peak amplitude and π is the constant 3.142.

where kilo means a unit of a thousand).

A tuning fork that produces the note 'A' commonly used for tuning musical instruments, vibrates at a frequency of 440 Hz. The note an octave above this vibrates twice as fast, at a frequency of 880 Hz, while the octave below has a frequency of 220 Hz. Human ears are sensitive to vibrations in the range of 20 Hz to 20 kHz (i.e. 20,000 cps), although at the ends of this range the note has to be very intense to be heard. Frequencies higher than 20 kHz are termed 'ultrasonic'. The frequency ranges of dogs and cats overlap with ours, but, unlike us, they can hear frequencies higher than 20 kHz.[2]

The measurement of phase relates to the stage in the cycle of vibration relative to a fixed point in time. Two sine waves of the same frequency and amplitude can be at different phases relative to each other. The cycle of vibration can be divided into 360 degrees. If there is zero phase difference the two waves will combine together to give one wave of twice the amplitude. If there is a phase difference of 180 degrees, then the two waves will cancel each other completely.[3] What this means, for a sound in air, is that any particular air molecule is being pushed in opposite directions by the same amount with the result that no vibration occurs, and hence no sound is heard. At other phase angles (besides multiples of 180 degrees) the resultant wave will be of intermediate amplitude. If the two waves differ slightly in frequency then this can be treated as a continually varying phase difference between waves of the same frequency and the result is a continually varying change of amplitude. The rate of this change is called the beat frequency and depends on the difference in frequency between the two primary waves. When the difference is large the beat frequency is high, when the difference is small the beat frequency is low. Perceptually beats are heard as a note of fixed frequency that changes in amplitude at a rate dependent on the frequency difference. The existence of the beat frequency can be put to practical use, as, for example, in tuning musical instruments.

The amplitude measure refers to the maximum extent of the vibration and this determines the intensity of a sound. The instantaneous amplitude varies sinusoidally (see Figure 2.1).

It is difficult to obtain a measure of sound intensity directly and instead the variation in sound pressure of the air molecules at a particular place is used. Pressure (measured as dynes per square centimetre or Newtons per square metre) can be used to determine intensity (measured as watts per square centimetre), since it is known that intensity is proportional to the square of pressure.

The decibel measure

The range of sounds of different sound pressure that the ear can respond to is so great (i.e. a range of 120,000,000 to 1), that units of sound pressure are not directly used. Instead the logarithmic measure of a decibel is used to express sound pressure or intensity. Firstly a ratio of a reference sound pressure (approximating to a sound at human hearing threshold) to the pressure produced by the sound source of interest is calculated, and this ratio is squeezed into more manageable units by obtaining the logarithm of the ratio. This unit is called a bel, in honour of Graham Alexander Bell the inventor of the telephone. However the bel is a large unit and the unit of a decibel, dB (1/10 of a bel) is more commonly used. The equation used to determine the decibel sound pressure level (dB SPL) of a sound is given below.

$$\text{dB SPL} = 20 \log_{10} \frac{\text{(root mean square sound pressure)}}{\text{reference pressure}}$$

The reference pressure used is 2×10^{-5} Newtons/square metre. (This reference pressure is equivalent to an intensity reference of 10^{-16} watts per square centimetre.)

A table of common sounds and their decibel values is shown in Table 2.1.

In practice the decibel level dB SPL of a sound is read directly from a scale on a sound level meter. The sound level meter will also have a weighting circuit so that dB(A) readings can be obtained. The dB(A) measure, as distinct from plain dB sound pressure level (dB SPL), includes a weighting that corresponds to the frequency sensitivity or frequency response of the ear, and is therefore a more relevant measure when considering the effect of a sound on human listeners. A method of determining the frequency response of the ear is described below, but it is important to realise that the human ear is more sensitive to frequencies in the range 1 to 5 kHz than to frequencies outside this range. Frequencies below 20 Hz would be felt rather than heard, while frequencies above 16 kHz have to be made very intense in order to be heard. Because very high frequency sounds (above 20 kHz) are outside the human frequency range, the contribution to overall sound pressure by these frequencies is

Table 2.1: Decibel values for common sounds

Sound	Approximate dB(A) level
Jet aircraft taking off	125
Loud orchestra	100
Thunder-clap overhead	90
Shouted speech	80
Manual typewriter	70
Normal conversation	60
Whisper	40
Quiet rural area at night	20

Note: The levels given are only approximate and apply to a listener in the local vicinity of the sound source. The sound intensity would decrease with distance from the source according to an inverse square law for most of these sounds.

ignored by the dB(A) measure. However, frequencies to which we are the most sensitive (in the range 2 to 4 kHz) are given the most weight. The dB(A) measure therefore attempts to take into account the frequency response of the ear and is usually more appropriate for assessing the effect of a sound on the human ear than the dB SPL measure, which treats all frequencies as equivalent.[4]

Most of the sounds in Table 2.1 are of a sustained or continuous nature and it is appropriate for the meter to record a value averaged over a period of time. For short sharp sounds (transients) such as explosions or impact sounds, however, the use of an average value to describe these sounds would be misleading, since these sounds have high peak values far in excess of the average value. The damage produced by these sounds is mainly due to the sudden rise and extent of sound pressure change, which may only last for a fraction of a second. To cater for this situation the dB meter can be set to record these peaks, and a peak reading together with an average reading is often quoted when describing sounds of this nature.

Decibel levels can cause some confusion when trying to use them to make loudness estimates, so as a rough guide it can be said that an increase in 3 dB of a sound will be just noticeable, while an increase of 10 dB will usually be heard as a doubling of loudness. Also, if two sounds of the same dB value are presented together, then there is an overall increase of 3 dB and not a doubling of the value (i.e. adding (or mixing) two sounds of 40 dB gives a result of 43 dB not 80 dB). Basically this is because it is the *sound pressure* that is added and the decibel value is the logarithm of this result. Note also that two tones of the same frequency and opposite phase would cancel completely.

If two sounds that differ by 10 dB or more are added, then the effective dB level would be that of the higher value of the two sounds (i.e. 80 dB plus 40 dB would still give an effective dB level of 80 dB).

The sound spectrum

In Figure 1 the sine wave is shown as a pattern in time, that is of a change of amplitude with time. There is, however, an alternative representation of sounds and vibrations that is in terms of a frequency spectrum. The sine wave of Figure 1 would appear as a line at a frequency of 1000 Hz or 1 kHz of a fixed amplitude. The length of the line indicates the amplitude. For sinusoids there might not appear to be much advantage to this alternative representation, but for complex sounds the frequency spectrum can be much easier to interpret than the time representation. Several sinusoids added together can produce a complex time waveform and it would in general be difficult to tell which sinusoids were present. The frequency representation, however, can tell you at a glance which frequency components are present, and also the amount of each component. Each frequency component would be represented by a sharp peak and the amount of that component would be indicated by the height of that peak. This is shown in Figure 2.2, in which a number of sounds are shown in both time and frequency representations.

It should be noted that click or transient sounds have a spectrum that is continuous, that is where the energy is distributed throughout the auditory range. Periodic sounds like pure tones and musical chords have discrete spectra, that is lines or sharp peaks at a particular frequency or frequencies. Non-periodic sounds such as hissing or a 'shush' noise have energy that is distributed fairly evenly throughout the auditory range. Noise that has equal power at any frequency is called 'white noise'.

The hearing threshold and frequency response of the ear

So far we have looked at how we can measure physical aspects of sounds. The sine wave or pure tone can now be used to characterise the hearing system. One important characterisation of any sound

19

Figure 2.2: Time amplitude waveforms and frequency spectra

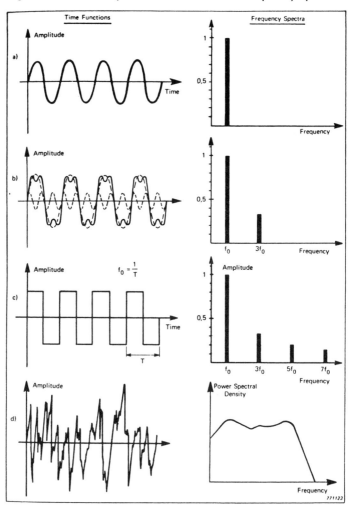

Time amplitude waveforms and frequency spectra of some simple sounds. (a) Is a pure tone or sine wave. (b) Two tones where the higher frequency tone is three times the frequency of the lower tone. (c) A square wave, which is composed of a fundamental frequency and the odd harmonics of decreasing amplitude. (d) White noise, which is a random signal having equal energy at all frequencies. (This is analogous to white light and the visible spectrum. In practice the energy falls off at the higher frequencies depending on the frequency response of the microphone.) (Adapted from figure 2.24 Sound signals and their Spectra. From 'Application of B & K Equipment to Acoustic Noise Measurements' by J.R. Hassel and K. Zaveri, Brüel and Kjaer.

Figure 2.3: Hearing threshold and equi-loudness curves

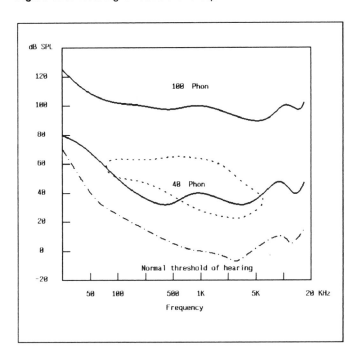

The figure shows the normal hearing threshold and the 40 phon and 100 phon equi-loudness curves (see text). The dotted 'contour' line indicates the region predominantly occupied by a speech signal in normal conversation.

system is its frequency response. That is how the system responds to tones of different frequency and intensity. For the ear the *threshold* frequency response may be found by finding the lowest intensity at which a sine wave, sometimes called a test or probe tone, of a particular frequency can be reliably detected (usually this means meeting a criterion of 75 per cent correct decisions concerning the presence or absence of the probe tone). The hearing threshold curve is constructed by repeating this measure for different frequency values of the sine wave. This is shown in Figure 2.3. Note that the threshold level for tones below 500 Hz and above 5 kHz becomes increasingly high as the tonal frequency is moved away from these values.

Figure 2.3 also shows a number of different curves demonstrating

21

a change in frequency-response with the overall level of the probe tone. Basically the frequency response curve becomes flatter as intensity is increased. These curves are known as equi-loudness curves. An equi-loudness curve is determined by setting a standard tone (usually at 1 kHz) to a particular level (dB SPL) and then adjusting the level of comparison tones of different frequencies until a match in loudness is achieved. The loudness measure of the phon is based on equi-loudness curves, and is basically the dB SPL value of a 1 kHz tone that is judged to be as loud as the target tone or sound. The 40 phon curve therefore indicates the dB SPL value at which any particular frequency in the auditory range sounds as loud as a 1 kHz tone at 40 dB SPL. For example, a 100 Hz tone at 50 dB SPL sounds as loud as a 1 kHz tone at 40 dB SPL, whereas to sound equally as loud a 4 kHz tone need only be at a level of 34 dB SPL.

There are two important features of these equi-loudness curves. First the difference in loudness of tones of equal intensity is greatest at threshold levels. This means that the rate of growth of loudness of tones with increasing intensity differs with tone frequency, being more rapid at low and high frequencies. This in turn means that a complex sound with a number of widely spaced frequency components will change in nature as the overall intensity is changed. This is a good reason for listening to orchestral music at intensity levels close to the original performance, since at lower intensities the tonal balance will suffer.

Threshold shifts

The effects of exposure to sustained intense sounds are reflected in a shift in the auditory threshold. The extent of such shifts and the recovery to normal threshold values have been studied (Hirsh and Ward 1952, Ward et al. 1958) in relation to the intensity, duration and frequency of the fatiguing stimulus. When the threshold returns to the previous value the shift is known as a temporary threshold shift (TTS). Long exposures can lead to a permanent shift (PTS). The form of the recovery curve often shows an initial improvement followed by a subsequent increase in the threshold at about an interval of two minutes after the fatiguing stimulus is turned off. This is known as 'bounce' in the recovery curve. The amount of threshold shift depends on the frequency of the tone used to determine the threshold and the frequency of the fatiguing stimulus. For intense stimuli the threshold shift is greater for frequencies above the fatiguing stimulus, being greatest for a frequency separation of one half-octave. A PTS obviously indicates permanent damage and this may also, as a consequence, produce tinnitus that has a pitch which correlates with the frequency at the edge of the damaged region.

PSYCHOLOGICAL ATTRIBUTES OF SOUNDS: PITCH, LOUDNESS AND TIMBRE

How does the ear 'measure' and compare sounds? When a simple tone such as a sinusoid is varied in frequency within the human hearing range there is a related change in the perception of that sound: the predominant change is one of pitch. Low-frequency sinusoids produce a low or deep pitch, and as frequency is increased then the pitch also increases. The loudness curves in Figure 2.3 indicate that loudness may also change when the frequency is changed, but pitch refers to the perception independent of the loudness change.

Complex sounds can also be periodic. The addition of a number of sine waves will produce a complex wave that is also periodic. In fact, Fourier's celebrated theorem tells us that any periodic wave can be analysed into a series of sine waves of the appropriate frequency, amplitude and phase. These periodic sounds will also usually have a distinctive pitch. Sounds that have predominant low-frequency components have a low pitch (e.g. the bass notes of a piano) while sounds with predominant high-frequency components have a high pitch (e.g. treble notes). This is not always the case, however, some complex sounds for example give a sensation of low pitch even when only medium to high frequencies are present. How the ear assigns a pitch to a complex wave partly depends on the periodicity of the sound and also the pattern of the prominent frequency components, including combination tones introduced by non-linear behaviour of the ear. The exact manner in which this happens is still a matter of debate, and this point will be discussed later in this chapter.

One term that is used in connection with complex sounds, particularly with musical instruments, is timbre. This refers to the pattern of harmonics that are produced by a sound source. Different musical instruments producing the same note are usually distinctive and while the note has the same pitch the timbre is different. Each instrument produces the same fundamental note but the presence and amount of the harmonics (whole multiples of the fundamental frequency, sometimes termed overtones) vary.

How does the ear make sense of sounds, particularly complex sounds such as speech and music? The complete answer is not yet available but there is a good deal of information about how simple sounds are processed by the ear and it is possible to suggest how more complex sounds may be processed in the light of this information. Perhaps the best way to achieve this is by first describing the parts of the ear and then by detailing their action and function in sound processing.

THE PARTS OF THE EAR

The overall structure of the human ear can be seen in Figure 2.4.

The first point of interest that a sound meets in the auditory pathway is the external ear or pinna. In dogs and cats the pinna is movable and this can help to locate the sound. In humans the ability to move the pinna is absent, however the pinna does help in localising sound. Experiments have shown that if the shape of the pinna is distorted or the hollows filled with wax then sound localisation can be impaired (Batteau 1967). The pinna is used primarily for locating the source of high-frequency sounds that have a wavelength which is less or of the same order of size as the pinna. Longer wavelengths from low-frequency sounds would 'bend round' the pinna so that their direction would be difficult to determine. High-frequency sounds (short wavelengths) are less susceptible to bending or diffraction by objects in the sound path, and hence are more useful for localisation purposes. This is one of the reasons that the drums in a marching band are heard before the band has turned the corner of the street, while the pipes are generally only audible when the band is in sight.

After the sound has entered the ear, the sound then travels down the auditory canal to the ear drum. The pinna together with the ear canal comprise the outer ear. The length of the canal is approximately 3 cm. Any tube closed at one end will resonate at a frequency at which the wavelength of the sound is related to the length of the tube (length of tube = ¼ wavelength of resonant frequency). For example, if you blow over the mouth of a bottle the air trapped in the bottle will resonate. The resonant frequency can be changed by altering the length of the air inside the bottle by pouring in some liquid. The resonant frequency in the case of the ear canal would be about 3 kHz. The situation is a little more

Figure 2.4: The external, middle and inner ears in man

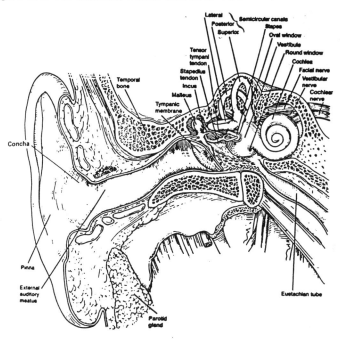

The figure shows a cross-section through the human ear. The outer ear is made up of the pinna and ear canal (external auditory meatus). The middle ear comprises the ear drum (tympanic membrane) and the ossicles, and like the outer ear is normally air-filled. The inner ear consists of the fluid-filled cochlea, semi-circular canals and the cochlear nerve. From 'Tissues and Organs: A Text-Atlas of Scanning Electron Microscopy' by Richard G. Kessel and Randy H. Kardon. Copyright © 1979, W.H. Freeman and Company.

complicated than the case of a simple tube because of the shape and position of the concha (the flap just in front of the ear canal). The consequence of this is that a band of frequencies over a mid-frequency range of 3 to 5 kHz are amplified.

The sound now reaches the ear drum (tympanic membrane) and causes this to vibrate. The size or amplitude of these vibrations is of some interest since at hearing threshold levels the amplitude of vibration is incredibly small, i.e. of the order of the diameter of a hydrogen atom. The vibrations are now transmitted through a mechanism of three small bones (ossicles), the hammer, anvil and stirrup (malleus, incus and stapes). The malleus is attached to the ear drum while the stapes terminates on the oval window membrane

25

of the cochlea and causes this to vibrate. The ear drum and the ossicles comprise the middle ear, which is air-filled via the eustachian tube. The eustachian tube is important since it serves to equalise the air-pressure on either side of the ear drum. It is normally closed, so that sudden changes in outside air-pressure, as in a climbing or descending aircraft, may cause pain. However, the eustachian tube is usually easily opened by chewing or swallowing motions, and the air-pressure in the outer ear and middle ear will then become equalised. If the eustachian tube is blocked because of a cold it may not be possible to equalise the pressure and then the ear drum may burst. This is the reason why it is not advisable to travel in light aircraft or to go under-water swimming with a head cold.

The oval window is the entry point to the inner ear, which consists of the fluid-filled cochlea, semi-circular canals and the cochlear nerve. Part of the job of the middle ear is to facilitate the transition from sound vibrations in air to vibrations in fluid, since the cochlear fluid would present a high impedance to air-molecule vibration. Without the middle ear, the impedance mis-match would result in most of the sound 'bouncing back' from the oval window instead of passing through. The middle ear, by virtue of the action of levers of the ossicles and the difference in size of the ear drum and oval window, amplifies the vibration and reduces the impedance mis-match, and so aids the passage of sound into the fluid-filled cochlea. The overall amplification of vibrations, from the ear drum to the oval window, introduced by the middle ear, is of the order of 18:1.

The ossicles do have other functions in that they can give a measure of protection to prolonged intense noise. A loud noise will usually initiate a reflex by the auditory system whereby the small muscles attached to the ossicles are activated. This then affects the mode of vibration of the ossicles so that the stapes twists rather than vibrates, which results in a reduction in movement at the oval window, thus giving some protection to the sensory cells within the cochlea. Unfortunately this reflex, known as the stapedius reflex, takes time to occur (10 to 20 milliseconds) and this is too slow to give protection against explosions, sonic bangs and sudden impact noises produced by most industrial machinery.

TRANSDUCTION: FROM MECHANICAL VIBRATIONS TO NEURAL IMPULSES

Once the sound enters the cochlea the process begins by which the pattern of vibrations is transformed and coded into a pattern of nerve impulses. A general term for this process is transduction. Inside the cochlea is an important structure called the basilar membrane. Figure 2.5 shows a cross-section through the cochlea and shows the relation of the basilar membrane to the organ of Corti, which contains the hair cells and tectorial membrane. There are two types of hair cell, the inner hair cell and the outer hair cell. There is one row of inner hair cells on one side of the arch of Corti and three rows of outer hair cells. In total there are about 25,000 hair cells in humans.

The cochlea itself is a small spiral structure of about two and a half turns, but for the purpose of understanding the way the sound is processed it can be rolled out as in Figure 2.6.

How could the cochlea act to discriminate sounds? One early theory, proposed by Helmholtz in 1857, was that the cochlea acted like a bank of tuned resonators (something like a scaled-down harp where the strings represent resonators of different frequency) and that a particular input frequency would cause the appropriate resonator to vibrate. Sensory cells attached to that resonator would 'tell the brain' which input frequency was present and sounds could be discriminated on the basis of the location of the active resonators on the cochlea. In this view each hair cell may be considered to be activated by a resonator. One problem with this theory is that the transverse sections of the basilar membrane are not 'taut' like the strings of a harp. This would imply that any resonators were highly damped, which would produce a poor selective frequency response. On the other hand if the resonators in the ear were lightly damped, which would mean a good selective frequency response, then the ear would continue to respond (this is known as 'ringing') long after the original sound had disappeared.

Another early theory, proposed by Rutherford in 1886, was that the cochlea acted like a telephone receiver. In this theory the basilar membrane (BM) would vibrate at the same frequency as the input tone and the sensory cells attached to the membrane would be 'switched on and off' at the input frequency. The brain was assumed to be capable of discriminating the rate of switching occurring in the auditory nerve. One problem with this theory is that it is known that the nerves attached to the sensory cells cannot represent high

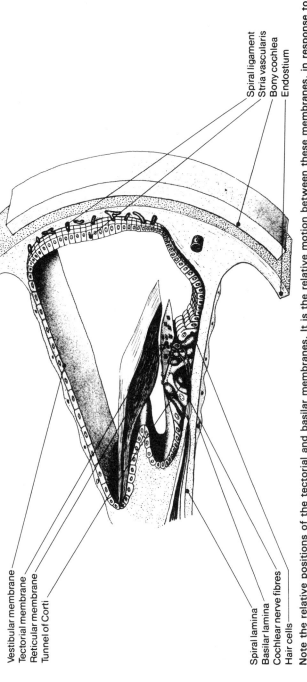

Figure 2.5: A cross-section of the cochlea showing the organ of Corti. From 'Serc in the treatment of Menière's Disease', Duphar Laboratories

Spiral ligament
Stria vascularis
Bony cochlea
Endostium

Vestibular membrane
Tectorial membrane
Reticular membrane
Tunnel of Corti

Spiral lamina
Basilar lamina
Cochlear nerve fibres
Hair cells

Note the relative positions of the tectorial and basilar membranes. It is the relative motion between these membranes, in response to sound, that provides the stimulus to the hair-cell that in turn produces activation of the nerve fibres and results in the perception of sound.

frequencies, that is they cannot switch on and off at rates much higher than a few hundred Hertz, so that most of the middle and high frequencies could not be encoded by this system. Since these early theories, important observations of the cochlea were made by von Bekesy (1928) and he also proposed a theory of cochlear action that has led to a better understanding of how the cochlear processes sound (a collection of his work can be found in von Bekesy, 1960).

Place theory of pitch perception

Bekesy's observations showed that when the stapes vibrates in the oval window the fluid vibrations produced in the cochlea act on the basilar membrane and set up a wave that travels along the length of the membrane. The direction and form of the wave is determined by the structure of the membrane, which differs in width and stiffness along the length of the cochlea. Basically the basilar membrane is narrower and stiffer at the oval window end (base end) and wider and less stiff at the top or apex of the cochlea. If a pure tone is stimulating the ear then the basilar membrane will vibrate at the same frequency. The travelling wave that is set up will produce amplitude displacements at different times along the basilar membrane. As the wave passes along the membrane there will be one place along the membrane at which the amplitude displacement is greatest. An envelope of displacement amplitudes can be drawn that shows this fact clearly (see Figure 2.6). For different frequencies of vibration the point of maximal displacement will exist at a different place. The high frequencies have their greatest amplitude at the oval window end and the low frequencies at the apical end. Frequencies can therefore be discriminated in terms of the place along the basilar membrane where displacement amplitude is greatest. If the ear can sense the point of maximal displacement, then a mechanism for responding to different frequencies is possible.

Attached to the basilar membrane are hair cells (in fact the basilar membrane is similar to a piece of skin with hairs). These hair cells make contact with the tectorial membrane, and are stretched and moved as the basilar membrane vibrates relative to the tectorial membrane. The greater the movement of the basilar membrane the greater the stimulation of the hair cells. This arrangement provides a mechanism for discriminating the frequency of vibration and of coding the frequency of periodic sounds.

To summarise, in Bekesy's theory, tones of different frequency

29

Figure 2.6: The cochlea and the Bekesy travelling wave

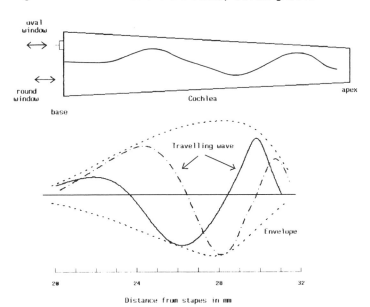

This figure shows a schematic representation of the cochlea and the position of the travelling wave set up on the basilar membrane in response to a pure tone (200 Hz), at two different times (corresponding to a phase separation of 90 degrees or $\pi/2$). The envelope represents the biggest displacement of the basilar membrane produced by the travelling wave at all positions on the basilar membrane. The peak of the envelope varies depending upon the frequency of the pure-tone stimulation. Low-frequency pure tones produce a peak in the envelope in the apical region of the basilar membrane while for higher frequencies the peak in the envelope occurs towards the base of the cochlea. The ear may therefore discriminate different frequencies according to the place of maximal displacement of the basilar membrane by the travelling wave. (Adapted from Bekesy (1960) *Experiments in Hearing*, McGraw-Hill, New York.)

will produce travelling waves that produce maximum displacement of the BM at different places along the basilar membrane. The hair cells will be stimulated the most at this place and thus frequency is coded in terms of the position of those hair cells that are responding the most to that input frequency. The overall amount of stimulation of the hair cells gives an indication of the intensity of the input zone.

Periodicity theory of pitch perception

There is another way in which the frequency or periodicity of a tone may be coded by the auditory system and this depends on the timing of the stimulation of the hair cells. The hair cell is thought to be stimulated every time the basilar membrane is deflected upwards. Stimulation of the hair cell leads to a generation of electric potential within the cell, which at a certain level causes the nerve fibre attached to the hair cell to 'fire'. That is, a spike discharge is initiated at the end of the nerve fibre (the synapse), which then travels upward along the auditory nerve. The spike has a number of interesting properties. First, it is an all-or-none event. If the hair cell is not sufficiently stimulated then the nerve firing does not take place. Second, the nerve spike is well defined in time and intervals between nerve firings could be measured to determine the stimulating frequency. The nerve firings are said to be 'phase-locked' to the stimulus, that is, there is a definite time-relation between the nerve firings and the stimulus waveform. The overall change from a mechanical pattern of vibration to a pattern of neural firings can also be seen as an analogue to digital conversion.

In this theory, the frequency or periodicity of a sound is coded in the periodicity present in the nerve firings, and it has, therefore, been termed the periodicity theory of hearing (Schouten 1940, 1970). For low frequencies (below 200 Hz or less), it would be possible for the hair cell to produce a nerve firing in its associated nerve fibre at the same rate as the input frequency. However, at higher input frequencies this cannot happen because there is a refractory period (a minimum period in which the nerve must 'recharge' itself before firing can occur again) in a nerve fibre, which lasts for about 20 milliseconds or so, just after the nerve has fired. This means that the auditory system must examine the periodicity present in a group of nerve fibres to code frequencies higher than a few hundred Hertz.

There is, however, an upper limit to the frequencies that can be encoded in terms of periodicity of nerve firings. This limit results from lack of absolute precision in the initiation of the nerve firing in response to the movement of the BM. There is always a slight random error or jitter in this process. For low frequencies the 'jitter error' is small compared with the period of the waveform but for higher frequencies the jitter time error is significant compared with the time-interval or period of the input wave. The highest frequency that could be encoded, in terms of nerve firing periodicity, is thought to be of the order of 5 kHz. Although this is well below the upper frequency limit of hearing it is known that the most important components of speech and music fall below this frequency limit (the telephone handset for example severely attenuates frequencies above 3 kHz).

The auditory system thus has a choice of ways to code frequency or periodicity in the input waveform and it is likely that both methods of coding are employed by the auditory system, although for high frequencies only a place encoding is possible. There is evidence from the ability to discriminate small frequency differences between pure tones that above 5 kHz this ability becomes markedly worse (Moore 1973). Such behaviour might be expected if the basis of pitch discrimination switched from a periodicity mechanism to a place mechanism.

The above description relates mainly to the analysis by the ear of simple sounds. For complex sounds, consisting for example of a number of frequency or spectral components, the problem is one of resolution. If a sound consists of two widely separated components in frequency, it is probable that the travelling wave displacement envelope shows two distinct peaks related to the two frequency components. If the position of these peaks is the same as if the two components were presented alone, then the system can resolve the frequency components. However if the two components are close together in frequency (within 5 per cent frequency difference) then the travelling wave displacement envelope is unlikely to show two distinct peaks and the components would not be resolved. In this situation a more powerful component might 'swamp' or 'mask' the weaker component.

MASKING

A consideration of the pattern of activation produced by the travelling wave on the basilar membrane suggests that low frequency tones will activate most of the hair cells attached to the basilar membrane while high frequency tones will not significantly activate hair cells in the apical (low frequency) end of the membrane.

This may explain why in the human auditory system it is easier to mask a signal tone with another tone (termed the masker) that is lower in frequency than the signal tone, rather than higher in frequency. This fact was initially reported by Mayer in 1876.

Figure 2.7: Masking effect of a tone

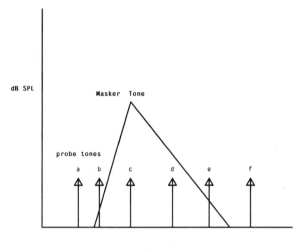

A simple representation of the masking effect of a tone is shown as a triangular pattern on the frequency axis (this may be roughly equated with the travelling wave envelope on the basilar membrane or the pattern of activation in the primary auditory nerve). Low-intensity probe tones are shown at different frequencies (a–e). In this representation the probe tone would be masked if it is completely within the triangular pattern produced by the masker tone (c and d). The tones at b and e frequencies would be partially masked, whilst the probe tones at a and f would be unaffected. The diagram indicates that the masker tone will mask more high frequencies than low frequencies.

Masking is most effective when the masker frequency components are close to the signal frequency (see Figure 2.7). As the frequency separation between signal and masker tone increases then the masker tone intensity has to increase in order to produce the same amount of masking. If white noise is used to mask a signal tone then only the frequencies in a band surrounding the tone are effective in masking. This band is sometimes known as a critical band and its size depends upon the signal frequency. The size of band increases as its centre frequency increases (Fletcher 1940; for a review of the work on critical bands see Scharf 1970). It is important to realise that masking can occur even though the masker sound and the signal do not overlap in time. When the masker occurs before the signal the process is called forward masking, and when the masker follows the signal in time, it is called backward masking.

Filters, and 'critical bands'

One way to discuss resolution and masking is to talk in terms of filters. A filter is a device that responds preferentially to certain items and rejects others. Usually the method of discrimination is in terms of a value on some dimension, e.g. size or in this case frequency of vibration. At any particular frequency one can imagine a filter positioned around that frequency. The width of the filter (or passband) is the range of frequencies around the central frequency that the filter passes (or responds to) without producing attenuation. An ideal rectangular filter would pass all frequencies within its passband without attenuation, but completely reject all other frequencies. Ideal filters, however, exist only in textbooks and a real filter is likely to have a rounded shape (see Figure 2.8).

The filter width can vary (width is usually quoted in octaves, e.g. 1/3 octave or 1/1 octave). Good frequency resolution would require filters of narrow bandwidths. If one component is to mask another then both components must lie within the filter passband (the range of frequencies responded to by the filter). In this respect the shape of the filter, as well as its bandwidth, is important. The shape of the auditory filter can be estimated by masking experiments in which the detectability of the signal is measured when it is sandwiched between two bands of noise and the frequency separation between the two noise bands is altered (Patterson 1976). It appears that the shape can be approximated by an inverted bell (or gaussian) shape.

One interesting property of filters is that good frequency resolution implies poor time resolution. (In order to know the frequency exactly an infinite amount of time is required.) There is a trade-off in frequency and time and any filter is a compromise between measuring these two values. The representation of the peripheral auditory system as a bank of filters does have some explanatory value. Damaged hearing can be described in terms of inactive filters or filters with abnormally wide bandwidths.

The term 'critical band' is often used to refer to a human auditory filter. More strictly a critical band is a frequency region within which different components are integrated or summed and outside of which the components act independently. Evidence for the critical band comes from threshold and loudness measurements of pure tones presented with varying frequency separation. The curves indicate that within a certain range of frequency separation there is no change in loudness or threshold of the two-tone complex as frequency separation is increased, but outside of this range there is an increase in loudness and an increase in threshold intensity.

Complex sounds may then be analysed by noting the pattern of output from a number of filters of different centre frequencies.

Non-linearity, distortion products and combination tones

A linear system is one in which the output follows changes in the input in a direct way, i.e. if the input is doubled then the output is doubled. Also, if two different input signals are combined then the output to the combined input should be the same as adding the outputs from the two individual inputs when they are presented alone. That is, no new frequency components are created, or put another way the whole is the sum of its parts. In general, the ear behaves in a linear fashion, however, in certain situations the ear does behave in a non-linear fashion and as a result new components are created that are perceptible and that are not present in the input to the ear. As with most pieces of measuring equipment there is a limit to the amount that can be measured and beyond which false readings are produced. The ear is no exception, so that with high-intensity sounds for which the ear cannot continue to increase its response to an increase in the input signal, distortion products and combination tones are produced. The difference tone is one example. If the input to the ear consists of two intense tones of frequencies f1 and f2, then the difference tone, the frequency of which is the difference between the two input frequencies $(f2-f1)$, may be heard as well. This is an instance where the ear perceives a component that is not present in the external world. The difference tone is only usually present when the input tones are intense, but other components or combination tones, such as a component at the frequency $(2f1-f2)$ may be heard when the input or primary tones are at medium intensities.

The missing fundamental

It has been known for some time that the pitch of complex tones may not correspond to any of the frequencies or components making up that complex tone. This observation has generated considerable interest among researchers because of its bearing on theories of pitch perception. For example, the spectrum of a pulse train (a series of pulses that are regularly spaced in time) is made up of a fundamental

Figure 2.8: The action of a filter

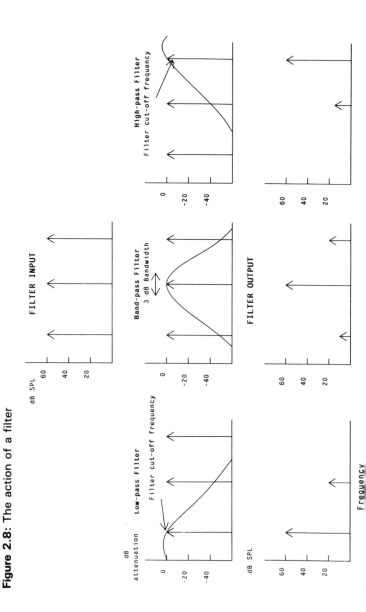

A schematic representation of the action of three types of filter (low-pass, band-pass and high-pass) on an input signal consisting of three tones is shown. It can be seen that the frequency response of the low-pass filter is such that the low-frequency tone magnitude is unaffected while the mid- and high-frequency tones are attenuated. A similar action is produced by the high-pass filter except it is the low-frequency tone that is attenuated the most. The frequency response of the band-pass filter shows that at the centre frequency the tone is not attenuated but that as the frequency decreases or increases there is progressively more attenuation. The 3 dB (or half power) bandwidth is the frequency range around the centre frequency outside of which attenuation is greater than 3 dB. Many different filter shapes are possible and it should also be noted that a filter will also affect the phase of a component as well as its magnitude.

component plus harmonics. The strongest component is usually the fundamental and it is not too surprising that the pitch of the signal also closely corresponds to the frequency of the fundamental. However, with some pulse trains (where the train is made up of pulses and alternate pulses are slightly displaced in time) the fundamental is no longer the strongest component and yet the pitch still corresponds to the fundamental frequency (Seebeck 1841). Further, if a fundamental frequency is removed by filtering, the pitch remains unaltered. This happens naturally with the low-frequency notes of a piano played softly. At such intensities the fundamental component would be below the hearing threshold and yet the pitch of the note stays the same. How could this be explained? The place theory has some difficulty in explaining this phenomena. An early suggestion was that the fundamental frequency was reintroduced into the ear by a non-linearity in the middle-ear. Although this is feasible at high intensities the phenomena also occurs at medium and low intensities. Also, if a band of masking noise that covers the spectral region in the vicinity of the fundamental is added to the complex tone again the pitch of the tone remains unaltered even though the presence of any component in this region would not be detected.

The periodicity theory of pitch perception does have a ready explanation in that if a number of harmonics all fall within one filter (see Figure 2.8) they beat together to produce a time-pattern the envelope of which reflects the fundamental periodicity of the complex tone. If nerve firings were initiated at local peaks within the envelope then the periodicity in these firings would be close to the period of the fundamental component. This mechanism may give rise to the pitch of complex tones.

Another possibility is that the pitch of complex tones is the result of pattern processing by the auditory system and that the pitch may be triggered even though part of a pattern (as when the fundamental is weak or filtered) is missing, since enough of the pattern, e.g. the harmonics, is still present.

Whatever the answer, it is clear that both the filtering action of the cochlear mechanics and the temporal representation in the timing of the neural firings are of great importance in the processing of signals by the auditory system.

THE AUDITORY PATHWAY

Further processing of the sound takes place as the neural firing pattern moves upwards along the auditory pathway. The main features of this pathway are shown in Figure 2.9.

It can be seen that the pathway is made of a number of 'stations' or nuclei, e.g. cochlea nucleus and superior olive, and that there is communication between the left and right sides of the pathway and also descending (called centrifugal) pathways from the cortex down to the cochlea. Like the visual system there appears to be a general principle of hierarchical organisation whereby units of the upper nuclei respond to complex stimuli (e.g. speech sounds) whereas at the lower levels the units respond to simple stimuli (e.g. pure tones). The purpose of the centrifugal pathways is still uncertain but these fibres can have both an excitatory and inhibitory effect on the cochlear nucleus, which allows the possibility of both simple attenuation of the ascending signal and possibly 'tuning' the peripheral units for improved signal-to-noise ratios.

One of the most important features is the neural communication between the ears, a phenomenon indicating that the inputs to the ears are compared. The comparison (or correlation of inputs to both ears) provides information as to the location of the sound and also helps in sorting out the signal from background noise and echoes. Comparison of the two inputs to the ears reveals two major differences. The first is an intensity difference that exists for a sound located to one side of the head. The head has a shadowing effect on the sound so that an intensity difference at the two ears gives a clue as to the position of the sound source. The second cue is in the arrival time of the sound. A brief sound, like a click, is well defined in time and if the sound source is positioned to one side of the head

Figure 2.9: The auditory pathway

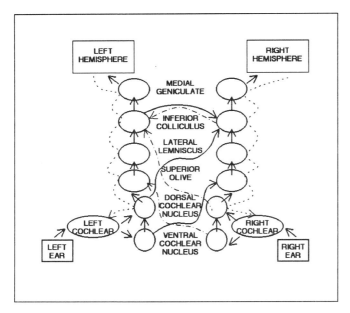

A schematic representation of the auditory pathway. The major
ascending pathways from the ear to the auditory cortex are shown. The
existence of descending (centrifugal) pathways is indicated by the dotted
lines.

the difference in arrival time of the sound at the two ears could be
used to locate the sound.

Although there are a number of positions that would give the
same time and intensity differences, small movements of the head
(or sound source) are sufficient to 'pin-point' the sound source
precisely. The ear can also make use of phase differences at the two
ears to locate non-transient sustained periodic sounds, e.g. sine
waves, provided that the half-wavelength of tone is greater than the
width of the head. For humans this means an upper limit of around
750 Hz.[5]

One interesting fact concerning binaural hearing is that it is
possible to add noise to one ear that will 'uncover', in the other ear,
a signal that is buried in the same noise. The ear obviously compares
the two inputs to the ears and decides that there is something
different, namely the signal, between them. How it does this is not
clear, but this observation emphasises that considerable binaural

processing is carried out by the auditory system.

Knowledge of the sound location is important for speech communication since it can improve the speech-to-noise ratio by 'tuning' in to a particular position. This is illustrated by our ability to listen to one particular conversation among many other ongoing conversations and also to switch between conversations. The way that the auditory system accomplishes this is not yet known and has been termed the 'cocktail-party' effect. Poor hearing in one ear impairs this ability, and while listening to one voice alone presents little problem, the introduction of other noises or other voices unfortunately has a drastic effect on speech perception.

This chapter has given a brief overview of the normal auditory system and it can be seen to be a complex and delicate mechanism. In the normal ear there is often a period of self-produced noise, hiss or whine, although this is usually short-lived and at low levels. However one of the consequences of damage is that the ear may generate a continuous noise and this is the condition known as tinnitus. Damage to the system can occur in many different ways and at different sites within the system.

Ways in which the site of lesion may be detected, and the manner in which tinnitus is generated are discussed in Chapters 4 and 5.

NOTES

1. Very low frequencies may only repeat or cycle in a period of several seconds, e.g. a frequency of 0.1 Hz would have a period of ten seconds. This frequency would not be heard but a fractional difference may be detected in some frequency ranges, e.g. the difference between 440 Hz and 440.8 Hz may be of some concern to musicians when they are tuning their instruments.

2. Dogs and cats are much more sensitive to these higher frequencies, partly because some of their natural prey, mice and rats, make high-frequency sounds.

3. The phase angle is often quoted in radians rather than degrees; 180 degrees is π radians. π is the ratio of the circumference to the diameter of a circle and can be approximated by the figure 3.142.

4. Usually other weighting circuits are available, e.g. dB(B) and dB(C); these measures attempt to account for the different shape in the equi-loudness curves as overall level is increased. The dB(A) measure is derived from the 40 phon equal-loudness curve while the dB(B) relates to the 70 phon curve and the dB(C) measure to the 100 phon curve. The phon measure and a way of determining an equi-loudness curve are described in Figure 2.3.

5. At frequencies higher than this the phase difference becomes ambiguous

since it may be due to a fraction of one wavelength or multiple half-wavelengths plus this same fraction. In practice useful phase difference cues can be obtained up to 1500 Hz, provided head movements are used to resolve ambiguity.

3

Definitions, Causes and Theories
of Tinnitus

DEFINITIONS

A basic broad definition of tinnitus would be the situation where there is a sensation of sound experienced by the tinnitus sufferer but there is no corresponding sound in the acoustic environment. The implication is that the sensation is mistakenly being generated within the hearing system itself or some noise or vibration is being produced nearby in the surrounding tissues or bones of the head. Stephens (1984) gives a full and very interesting account of the medical treatment of tinnitus, starting with the advice of the Assyrians and Mesopotamians in 700 BC! However, volume 19 of J.A.H. Murray's *A New English Dictionary*, published by the Clarendon Press in 1916, indicates that the first definition of tinnitus is to be found in a translation of Blancard's *The Physical Dictionary* (ed 2) of 1693 as: '*Tinnitus Aurium* — a certain buzzing or tingling in the Ears'. The words derive from the Latin *tinnire* meaning to ring or tinkle and *auris* referring to the ear. The current *Oxford English Dictionary* defines tinnitus as a sensation of ringing in the ears. Other early references noted by Murray are to an article by R.J. Graves in *System of Clinical Medicine* (*xiv*, p. 170), published in 1843, in which someone is said on admission [to hospital] to have 'complained of headache, tinnitus aurium'. A later reference cited is in *St. George's Hospital Report* (*IX*, p. 649) of 1879, in which note is made of 'the development of constitutional symptoms such as tinnitus and slight deafness'.

Well over 100 years ago, then, medical papers were being written that discussed drugs in the treatment of tinnitus (muriate of ammonia, nitrate of silver, nitrate of amyl) as well as the effect of electrical current (galvanic current). However, the Third Serial of the Surgeon-General's Index Catalogue, published in 1932, contains entries for only 29 publications concerning tinnitus. Whether this reflects a lessening of interest in the topic is unclear. What *is* clear is that *objective* forms of tinnitus were well known — i.e. forms of tinnitus in which a noise could be heard by persons other than the individual with tinnitus. This brings us to the first sub-classification of tinnitus into *subjective* types, which apparently can only be heard by the person with tinnitus, and *objective* types, which may be audible to others as well.

In subjective tinnitus, the neural signals corresponding to the tinnitus, which are present in the auditory cortex, may have been produced by a lesion in the cortex itself, or at any further stage in the auditory pathway. The tinnitus, however, is usually 'heard' as a sound that is close to or at the ear.

An analogy of a lift may help explain this: imagine standing at the top of the building (the auditory cortex) when the lift arrives and discharges its passengers (neural signals, which are interpreted as being produced by sounds); there is no way of telling at which floor the passengers may have boarded the lift. The auditory cortex assumes that everybody got on at the ground floor, that is, all signals have an *origin* at the auditory periphery (or cochlea). This assumption is 'wired in' to the cortex since this is how the normal ear operates. The tinnitus signal may have in fact got on at the 'ground floor', as when the cochlea malfunctions and produces spurious signals. However, the tinnitus signal may have boarded at another 'floor' (e.g. the cochlear nucleus or superior olive or the medial geniculate in the auditory pathway, see Figure 2.8).

Subjective tinnitus is, in a sense, an hallucination in that it is something perceived with no known external cause, but it is not an hallucination in the layman's understanding of the term — the latter is referred to by Longridge (1979) as *formed tinnitus*, when the sound is organised into patterns as in music or speech. The word hallucination suggests something that is not 'real'. The awful 'reality' of some forms of tinnitus is brought home by Aran and Cazals (1981, p. 217) when they suggest tinnitus may be viewed in some senses as a pain:

> Many analogies exist between pathological pain sensations — that is, pain sensations not caused by external excitation of receptors — and tinnitus. They are both hallucinations. They can profoundly disturb the affected patient. These sensations are strongly dependent on, and may alter, the psychological status of the patient. In the worst conditions they may lead to suicide. Indeed, subjective tinnitus, which may dramatically affect some

patients, is never as clearly 'objectifiable' as the reality of unbearable pain manifested by some patients with cancer. Yet we should not believe that subjective hearing sensations cannot be as strongly experienced as pathological pain.

Loavenbruck (1980) suggests a classification whereby the initial differentiation is made between tinnitus of *central* origin — i.e. the origin of it is thought to be due to malfunctioning of processes within the brain, or *peripheral* — i.e. the origin is considered to be outside or peripheral to the brain, usually in the ear or in the nerves from the ear to the brain. He refers to peripheral tinnitus as *tinnitus aurium*, whereas central tinnitus he labels *tinnitus cerebri*. He then subdivides peripheral tinnitus into *objective* and *subjective* types. Loavenbruck suggests that tinnitus cerebri, central tinnitus, is a non-localised, subjective sensation that is diffuse and non-specific. This seems to confuse the location of the noise with the likely location of its possible cause. According to Shucart and Tenner (1981, p. 166) the whole question of whether tinnitus is peripheral or central *in origin* is confusing. The border zone both for definition and treatment of tinnitus is poorly defined — 'which often leads to patients being shuttled among neurologists, neurosurgeons and otolaryngologists'. At present the classification of tinnitus as *central* or *peripheral* in terms of the location of the causative agent or agents would appear difficult to establish for a large proportion of tinnitus cases.

When no precise clinical (medical) diagnosis concerning tinnitus can be made and when it is a matter of conjecture where the causative damage lies, the tinnitus is often referred to as *idiopathic*.

CAUSES AND THEORIES OF TINNITUS

In this section we describe a number of known causes of tinnitus and also some theories and 'explanations' of the mechanism by which the tinnitus signal is generated. In some cases the level of explanation is detailed enough to include an account of how tinnitus arose and how it is sustained by the system, but other explanations merely describe a likely site for the generation of tinnitus. Perhaps the most easily identified and understood forms of tinnitus are those referred to by the term 'objective head noises'.

Objective Head Noises

The often-cited references to *objective* head noises are to the least frequently occurring forms of tinnitus but the most dramatic ones, usually those that can be heard relatively easily by others without the need to use stethoscopes or other forms of noise-amplifying instrumentation. All forms of objective head noises are rare, and Longridge (1981) suggests that they are present in only some 1 per cent of patients who have tinnitus as a main complaint. Nevertheless, Brennan and Salerno (1981) note that 'hums' associated with blood flow (venous hums) occur in all children and in 26 to 66 per cent of young adults — but these are rarely heard by the individual as tinnitus.

Dramatic examples

Glanville, Coles and Sullivan (1971) give an account of a family with high-tonal objective tinnitus. The young child of the family had a high-pitched tinnitus that could be heard at a distance of four feet. The child was teased at school because its ears 'sang'. The child's father and one of its siblings had similar but less-remarkable emissions, and the father could not hear his own noise. (This poses a definitional problem. If the person with the noise cannot hear it, should it be regarded as tinnitus, which is usually defined as the perception of noise, often without external cause?) McFadden (1982, p. 6) cites other sources, giving details of a girl whose ear emitted a high-pitched noise (also inaudible to her), as well as examples of objective tinnitus in animals. Aran, in a discussion that followed Douek's paper on the classification of tinnitus (1981) mentions a nine-year-old girl who had a small high-frequency hearing loss in both ears. By placing a microphone in the outer ear canal a clear high-pitched tone (8500 Hz, 30dB SPL) could be heard and recorded. As we shall see later, more sensitive microphones are more able to pick up such acoustic emissions.

Objective types of tinnitus

Virtanen (1983) suggests that objective tinnitus can be divided into the vascular and the muscular type. In the former an often high-pitched tinnitus is caused by abnormalities within the arteries of the head and neck or is due to an anomaly in the system of veins at the base of the skull. In the muscular-type — or click-type — tinnitus, the noise is caused largely by palatal myoclonus — rigid contractions of the muscles situated behind the back teeth. This sound is similar to the irregular ticking of an alarm clock or the noise caused by the snapping of two finger nails against one another. In at least one instance, that of the first author, it is known that such clicks can be produced voluntarily.

Myoclonus (muscle spasm)

Virtanen (1983) considered that hitherto, the source of the clicking sound was thought to be due to either the snapping together of the eustachian tube (the tube leading from the back of the throat to the middle ear, which helps maintain equal air pressure between the outer and middle ear), a rapid spasm of contractions and relaxations of one of the middle ear muscles (the tensor tympani), a similar spasm in another middle ear muscle (the stapedius muscle), or a wide-open eustachian tube (in the latter instance the individual may hear his own breathing magnified). All of these, says Virtanen, have to be differentiated in the diagnosis of palatal myoclonus, and Fernandez (1983) mentions a variety of techniques (tympanometry electromyographs and electroencephalographs that may help in establishing the diagnosis. Virtanen refers to *tubal* tinnitus as the sound heard when the walls of the eustachian tube snap together. (He also mentions that in cases that are very distressing, cutting of the tensor veli palatini muscle tendon may be a useful method of treatment.)

Venous and arterial hums

Perhaps the most common cause of this type of objective tinnitus arises from irregular or disturbed blood flow through the large arteries going to the head. Sounds arising from abnormalities in or abnormal communications between blood vessels in the neck or skull cavity may result in objective tinnitus. In this sense the tinnitus has little to do with the hearing system save that the system is hearing other internal sounds — mainly those in its own vicinity. These hums may often be heard through a stethoscope and are usually low-pitched and pulsatile in character (Chandler 1983). The tinnitus that arises from and within the internal jugular vein (a very large blood vessel carrying blood from the brain, running internally vertically down the side of the neck) is particularly important, since it is this type that may be loud enough to interfere with sleep and result in some loss of hearing. Chandler points out that a variety of things such as diseased widenings or bulges or weak spots in arteries, long sinuous ulcers or narrow pus-inducing canals, and small hard discoidal eruptions in veins and arteries can give rise to objective

46

tinnitus and states that, given their actual incidence as body noises, it is remarkable that venous hum tinnitus has been reported so infrequently in the otologic literature.

Other hums

It appears that certain low-frequency hums *are* due to objective internal head and neck noises although it was once hypothesised that persons hearing such hums might have super-sensitive hearing and might actually be hearing real low-intensity hums emanating from environmental sources (distant machinery, electricity sub-stations, telegraph wires, and such like). It is thought that venous hums may arise in veins and arteries that are *not* abnormal or diseased. It is possible that a viscous fluid like blood flowing through a flexible-walled tube, such as a vein or artery, may induce the walls to vibrate (Walford 1980). George, Reizine, Laurian, Riche and Merland (1983) and Hardison, Smith, Crawley and Battey (1981) report surgical forms of treatment for annoying noises arising from the dominant jugular vein, as do others (Brennan and Salerno 1981). The 'singing' ear of the child mentioned above was postulated to be produced by fibrous strands vibrating in the sigmoid or jugular blood flow (Hazell 1979a).

Spinal fluid pressure

Meador, Stefadouros, Malik and Swift (1982), reporting on a self-heard venous noise suggested it was directly due to increased pressure of the spinal fluid around the brain. When a device was arranged to reduce this pressure, the tinnitus, which had been a pulsatile whistling noise in the right ear, disappeared. The underlying cause is still likely to be some form of turbulence in the blood system, exacerbated by high spinal fluid pressure.

Shunts

Shunts are diversions, or new or unexpected or abnormal connections, those between the arterial and the venous blood systems sometimes being thought to give rise to tinnitus when occurring in close proximity to the hearing mechanism. Lind and Lundquist (1979) reported one such shunt that produced an objective tinnitus — a pulse-synchronous murmur — which could be recorded by microphones placed on the mastoid bones behind each ear. A technique for showing defects in blood vessels by means of X-rays (angiograms) revealed an unexpected connection between an artery at the back of the head and the sigmoid sinus. After surgical removal of these shunts on both sides of the head, the incapacitating tinnitus disappeared. Lind and Lundquist discuss the importance of making a thorough medical examination when pulse-synchronous tinnitus is in evidence, since in many cases there are effective surgical treatments for the condition.

Nerve compression

Lesinski, Chambers, Komray, Keiser and Khodadad (1979) suggest that nerve compression may also be one factor in the production of pulsatile tinnitus, although in this particular instance the tinnitus may be subjective even though the cause may be objective. They present evidence, again using X-ray examinations, showing how in three cases an artery (the trigeminal artery) took an unexpected route in which it crossed the nerve of hearing (the eighth nerve — the nerve carrying signals from the ear to the brain). In these cases it was suggested that pulsatile pressure by the artery on the eighth nerve was responsible for the pulsatile nature of the tinnitus.

Jaw joint noises

The medical adviser to the British Tinnitus Association points out, in a 'question and answer' session about tinnitus, that roughness in the jaw joint just in front of the ear may produce sounds that are audible as an objective form of tinnitus (BTA, 1980). Brookes, Maw and Coleman (1980) examined 45 patients with forms of jaw joint dysfunction, pain in the ear originating in a nerve, and other aural symptoms (such as tinnitus, deafness, pressure/blockage and dizziness with definite sensations of rotational movement) — sometimes referred to as Costen's syndrome. They concluded from their study that in 91 per cent of cases the aural symptoms were purely coincidental to the joint dysfunction. They considered this finding compatible with the relatively common occurrence of such aural symptoms and of jaw dysfunction in the general population. The one aural problem that did seem to be directly connected with jaw dysfunction was otalgia — *pain* in the ear originating in a nerve.

Subjective tinnitus

In the previous section we were mainly concerned with sounds generated within the head, but external to the auditory system, and which were received as an input to the inner ear. In the following section we are concerned with tinnitus that arises within the cochlea or in the subsequent stages of the auditory system.

In most cases of tinnitus there is also accompanying hearing loss indicating damage to the system, usually at the level of the cochlea and in particlar damage to the hair cells. Damage to the system may be the result of Menières Disease, acoustic trauma (resulting from very loud noises, such as explosions), long-term exposure to loud noise (factory workers are prone to such damage) and also the effects of ageing. Damage can also occur from the effect of drugs and certain diseases. In general terms, such damage would effect the normal operation of the cochlea leading to hearing loss and often also to tinnitus. How could this come about?

One possibility is that the hair cells become detached (decoupled) from the tectorial membrane and respond therefore not to the travelling wave located on the basilar membrane produced by external sounds, but instead to any movement of the cochlear fluids, possibly even to Brownian movement (random movement of fluid particles due to thermal energy). Brownian movement would be present at all times and might therefore explain the presence of tinnitus in the absence of other sounds. Tonndorf (1980) has argued that the 'noise-level' at the hair cell transduction phase will be increased by loss of stereociliary stiffness, that is in the tension of the hairs or cilia connecting the hair cell to the tectorial membrane. This is referred to as partial decoupling (rather than a complete separation between the hair cells and tectorial membrane). This view would suggest that a localised region of decoupling would produce a 'tonal' tinnitus, whereas widespread decoupling would give rise to a 'noise-like' tinnitus. It is possible that the tinnitus associated with Menière's Disease is produced by such a mechanism.

Menière's Disease

Menière's Disease is a disorder of the hearing and balance organs. The age of onset is usually between 30 and 60 years and affects males and females in about the same proportion. Tinnitus is one of three well known symptoms of Menière's Disease, the others being vertigo and a hearing loss (usually predominantly in the low-frequency region and of the order of 15 to 60 dB, which is accompanied by loudness recruitment). The disease was first described in 1861 by Menière. The onset of an attack of Menière's Disease (where all symptoms are present, including the debilitating symptoms of vertigo) can be sudden, but may be heralded by a feeling of fullness in the ear and by the symptoms of hearing loss and tinnitus for a day or two before the attack (House 1975). The attack of Menière's may last for several days and the associated vertigo may be of sufficient intensity to confine the sufferer to bed until the attack subsides. In the early stages of Menière's Disease the symptoms are reversible; and the use of Serc (beta histamine) is generally reckoned to be effective in reducing the frequency and severity of attacks of Menière's (Frew and Menon 1976). Menière's Disease is generally thought to be associated with a vascular disorder leading to an accumulation of endolymph in the cochlear duct. Recent work has suggested the mechanism by which the associated tinnitus could arise (Ylikoskij 1979, Dohlman 1980). In an attack of Menière's the build up of fluid within the inner ear continues until the increased pressure is relieved by a rupture of one of the cochlear membranes, usually the vestibular membrane. The hair cells are thus subject to two potentially damaging events. First, an increase of pressure that may affect the compliance of the hair cell or produce a partial decoupling of the hair cell from the tectorial membrane. As mentioned previously this would be expected to increase the noise level at the hair cell transduction stage and give rise to tinnitus. Secondly, the rupture of the vestibular membrane would disturb the ionic concentration gradient across the hair cell (the chemical battery necessary for the generation of the neural signals), which would result in desensitisation and loss of response of the hair cell to sound. The hair cells most affected are in the apical region of the cochlea, which is the region most responsive to low-frequency sound. This fact ties in with the observation that the tinnitus associated with Menière's Disease usually has a low pitch (often reported as a roaring noise). It may be that the tinnitus is generated mainly at the edge of the temporarily damaged region, and it would be of interest to obtain more information of the changes in the pitch, loudness and responsiveness to masking of the tinnitus, but as McFadden (1982) points out, a patient undergoing a Menière's attack is unlikely to be able to cooperate in such an experiment. However it is possible that such information may be gathered at a tinnitus clinic in the near future.

Spontaneous activity

Another possible cause of tinnitus is an increase in the spontaneous firing rate of the auditory nerve. In most neural systems there is always a certain background level of activity or noise that is uncorrelated with the sensory input. The spontaneous firing rate of auditory fibres varies from a few spikes per second to about 100 firings per second, although the fibres fall into two groups: a low spontaneous rate group (0 to 15) per second and a high spontaneous rate group (15 to 100) firings per second (about 75 per cent of fibres; Kim and Molnar, 1979). An increase in this spontaneous rate (above a certain threshold) may lead to a sensation of sound even when no external sound is present. The increase in spontaneous activity may result from a change in the local environment of the sensory receptor, e.g. blood supply or chemicals in the blood. It is known, for example, that high dosages of salicylate (aspirin) may produce tinnitus and temporary hearing loss when blood concentrations exceed 200 mg/l (Mongan *et al.* 1973). It has also been shown that salicylate can temporarily cause changes in the spontaneous activity in auditory nerve fibres (Evans *et al.* 1981). There is some debate on the effect of noise exposure on the spontaneous firing rate. In general, it appears that the effect of exposure to intense noise is to depress the spontaneous firing rate of fibres as well as to produce an elevation in threshold in the period following noise exposure. However some studies have reported an increase in the spontaneous firing rate (Liberman and Kiang 1978, Schmiedt *et al.* 1980).

Denervation hypersensitivity

In a hierarchically organised system as complex as the human auditory system, the neural signal generated at the cochlea undergoes several stages of processing before it reaches the cortex. For processing to occur, a nerve cell typically receives a number of inputs from primary receptor cells. These inputs may have an excitatory or inhibitory effect and the higher order cell may also receive excitatory or inhibitory inputs from its neighbours (or even from cells at higher levels, e.g. auditory cortex, so that feedback control is possible). Given this rich interconnection, all manner of processing is possible. However, it is quite feasible that damage to a peripheral stage may in fact lead to some cells at the cochlear level or at higher levels becoming more active or hypersensitive (this is sometimes known as denervation hypersensitivity). For example, if damage to peripheral cells resulted in the reduction of inhibitory input to a higher order cell, then that cell may in fact *increase* its output. In turn, this increase of activity may produce a sensation of a sound when in fact no external sound is present. It is possible that a similar situation may exist with some forms of tinnitus. Thus damage originally at the periphery could, because of the *reduction* in input, lead to the cortex becoming more active and producing tinnitus.

Central tinnitus

Although the subject may report the tinnitus as being at the ear, tinnitus may be centrally located much in the same way as phantom limb pain is felt as pain in the missing limb.

Martin (1982) considers that central brain processes are a component in some cases of persistent tinnitus because the primary condition known to be causing the condition can be cured, whereas the tinnitus may remain. Central processes also appear to influence the perception of tinnitus and one reason why often tinnitus seems louder on waking up is attributed to a central 'volume or sensitivity control' in the brain that 'turns up' the inner ear in conditions of quiet and during sleep.

Young and Lowry (1983) suggest that in some cases a permanent tinnitus may start in the ear *opposite* to that which has been exposed to intense sounds, and in a similar vein Shulman and Seitz (1981) suggest that, for example, a patient with right-sided tinnitus may have a generator site for it in the left ear.[1] As Hazell (1979a) points out, many cases of tinnitus must be due to a central auditory pathology because cutting the acoustic nerve from the ear to the brain or anaesthetising the cochlea in the inner ear fails in 50 per cent of cases to relieve the tinnitus (p. 470). Others suggest that even though the original damage is commonly in the ear — i.e. the damage is peripheral — there is a central *component*, and output from the brain to the ear (efferent signals) may play a part in causing it (Anon, 1979; Shulman, 1981a).

Vernon, in the final general discussion at the Ciba Foundation Symposium on Tinnitus (Evered and Lawrenson, 1981, p. 280) notes that patients given tinnitus masking devices for one ear frequently say that the masker stops the tinnitus in that ear and makes it more noticeable in the other ear. He suggests that this is some sort of centrally mediated 'contrast phenomenon'. In the same discussion, Evans (p. 282) suggests that the sorts of subjective tinnitus mostly studied may be caused by *both* central and peripheral factors. As far as this issue is concerned perhaps the situation is best summed up by Majumdar, Mason and Gibbin (1983, p. 175): 'Whilst tinnitus may accompany almost any otological disorder, its site of origin and the method of its development and generation are unknown.'

At present the site of causation of most forms of subjective tinnitus is a matter for speculation.[2]

Otoacoustic emissions and the 'cochlear echo'

For reasons that we will examine shortly, the classical division of tinnitus into subjective and objective forms has recently been complicated by the addition of another class of tinnitus sounds. In classical *subjective* tinnitus there are perceptions of sounds that have (as yet) no detected objective counterpart and that are presumably caused by abnormal activity at some place or places in the auditory nervous system. In classical *objective* tinnitus there are perceptions of sound that *do* have an objective, often vibratory, concomitant originating from some structure in the middle or inner ear or elsewhere in the head and neck. It has recently been discovered that there *are* sounds, apparently emitted by the cochlea in the inner ear, that are physically detectable in the ear canal at the entrance to the ear, but which are *not* necessarily audible to the individuals who have them. McFadden (1982, p. 7) goes on to suggest that:

Even more refined procedures may eventually reveal acoustic concomitants [i.e. ones that can be objectively detected as sound] of other forms of tinnitus, thereby moving them from the subjective to the objective category, and conceivably, non acoustic [i.e. nonaudible] but nevertheless objective measures of some forms of tinnitus may be developed that will further muddy the distinction between the objective and subjective forms of the malady . . .

It should be noted that a recent major publication on tinnitus [Ciba Foundation Symposium 85] explicitly proposes to exclude from the definition of tinnitus those cases previously classified as objective. While the objective/subjective distinction may have become muddy in recent times, and may deserve to be dropped, there is no apparent justification for disregarding history and tradition by excluding from the definition those 'head noises' that happen to have an acoustic concomitant.

Even more refined and complex classifications for tinnitus have been suggested by Shulman and Goldstein (1984) and by Ghosh (1978).

The objective forms of tinnitus outlined above arise largely from body noises in the environment around the hearing mechanism. However some noises are thought to be produced *by the ear itself* — probably from within the cochlea in the inner ear. These noises have been termed otoacoustic emissions (OAEs).

It is the discovery of these noises that has blurred earlier distinctions between objective and subjective forms of tinnitus. In some cases noises produced by the inner ear are not heard by the individual producing the noise, and in nearly all cases they can only be heard objectively by the use of ultra-sensitive microphones placed in the ear canal, which is sealed so that small pressure changes can be detected. The emissions that are detected consist of narrow bands of noise (about a 10 Hz bandwidth) localised at a constant centre frequency. The emissions can be masked and beats are heard if an external tone of similar frequency is presented. The emission is also suppressed following the presentation of an intense tone that is sufficient to cause a temporary threshold shift. When short durations of tones of frequencies below the emission frequency are used, there is suppression followed by a period of 'enhancement' or increase in the emission (Kemp 1981). This behaviour is similar to that of residual inhibition of tinnitus, where tinnitus can be markedly suppressed following a period of masking (see Chapter 5). Hazell (1981a) states that there is little reason to doubt that these sound emissions represent the spontaneous mechanical generation of sound energy within the cochlea. Tyler and Conrad-Armes (1982) report the results of placing such sensitive microphones in the ear canals of 20 subjects without subjective tinnitus and in those of 25 subjects reporting tinnitus. In five subjects without tinnitus, and in one with, spontaneous acoustic cochlear emissions were recorded (typically between 800 Hz and 2000 Hz, and at between 2 and 12 dB SPL). In the patient with tinnitus there was no clear relation between the pitch of the tinnitus (as determined by psychophysical matching) and the frequency range of the emission.

It is not yet clear whether such *spontaneous* emissions have the same origin as *evoked* emissions, i.e. those that can be produced by introducing a sound to the ear. These *evoked* emissions are usually known as cochlear *echoes* since it appears that the cochlea actively echoes back some of the sound put into it. The work of Kemp (1978) on the cochlear echo and subsequent work by Wilson (1980a,b) and Mountain (1980) has indicated that the transduction process in the cochlea (that is the change from mechanical motion on the cochlea partition to neural activity) cannot be treated as a purely passive linear process, but may involve an active component. The existence of a sustained cochlear echo and spontaneous acoustic emissions indicates that the stimulation of the hair cells by the mechanical movement of the basilar membrane can result in mechanical energy being fed back to the cochlea. The existence of feed-back in a system means that it is possible for a sensory system to continue to respond to a signal long after the original signal has disappeared, since the sensory system can 'excite' itself! Kemp (1980, p. iv) outlines his discovery of the cochlear echo, thus:

> Some years ago, whilst performing laboratory experiments on my own (normal) hearing, I became interested in the noises and distortions in my ears which I could hear only when in a very quiet room. Many 'normally hearing' people have these noises: often quite pure tones. After much research it proved possible to detect these sounds using a special miniature microphone fitted into the ear canal . . .
>
> The surprising thing was that when provided with sound, rather than silence, the healthy ear stepped up its own sound generation. It responded to sound by producing a faint but measurable echo of that sound . . .
>
> In making these discoveries we have explained for the first time one mild form of 'subjective' tinnitus. We call this 'cochlear oscillation tinnitus' and it seems to be a normal function of the ear out of control, i.e. 'feedback howl' [as when a microphone picks up too much of its own output from loudspeakers, or when a covered-up hearing aid 'whistles'] inside the ear.

Wilson (1980a) provides one model for explaining the length of time the 'echo' takes to appear, based on an hypothesis that the minute hair cells in the cochlea swell in volume at certain stimulus frequencies and subsequently contract. Wilson (1980b) also suggests that his findings support the view of Kemp, that acoustic re-emissions (i.e. the echo) and tinnitus and the fine-structure of hearing acuity are inter-related in some way, and in most instances originate within the cochlea in the inner ear. The fine-structure of hearing acuity reflects the ability of the individual to hear sounds at very low volumes at a multitude of frequencies. This often reveals peaks and troughs in acuity at different but quite particular frequencies. Conventional audiometers for measuring hearing often only measure the threshold — the minimum sound level at which a person hears the sound — at 10 different fixed frequencies (from low frequencies of 125 Hz to 'high' frequencies of 8000 Hz). Research instruments can measure threshold at *any* frequency and can thus detect precise frequencies or frequency ranges at which the hearing threshold might rise (showing less acuity at that point) and around which tinnitus as an objective sound emitted from the ear might also occur.

During many of the experiments Wilson (1980b) conducted, subjects reported hearing tones in some cases in the absence of stimulation and which in other cases were induced by noise stimulation and which interacted with it. Interestingly, in one experiment tinnitus was never reported by one subject when his body was upright and no objective emissions were detectable either; when in an inverted position, however, a continuous low tone could be heard that could be repeatedly and reliably stopped and started by taking the appropriate body position.

It would be convenient to hope that eventually most forms of *subjective* tinnitus would be found to have a counterpart in spontaneous acoustic *objective* emissions. As yet most spontaneous emissions that have been detected have been of a relatively low frequency, while much subjective tinnitus is high in pitch. For example, research by Zurek (1981), has generally failed to find spontaneous acoustic emissions in the ears of tinnitus sufferers and also in most cases failed to find a correspondence between 'tinnitus pitch' and spontaneous acoustic emissions when both are measurable in the tinnitus sufferer. Also Rutten (1980) who looked for OAEs in both normal-hearing and hearing-impaired groups found that the emissions were most common in the normal-hearing group.

In the case of tinnitus of medium to high pitch this might simply reflect the experimental difficulties inherent in recording emissions higher in frequency than 3 kHz, because of the transmission characteristics of the middle ear (which would act as a low-pass filter). McFadden (1982) considers that while it is disappointing to many who had momentarily hoped that some forms of hitherto subjective tinnitus would, in the event, prove to be objective, and hence more easily studied and perhaps, even, more easily treated, it appears on current evidence that otoacoustic emissions will not prove responsible for many instances of severe, problem tinnitus.

NOTES

1. They suggest that from the point of view of effective masking it may be better to put the masker on the generator site ear (where known) rather than in the ear in which the noise appears to the patient to be.

2. Many researchers argue for a central 'component' in 'peripheral' tinnitus (Lackner 1976, Johnson and Mitchell 1984, Tyler 1984, Tyler and Conrad-Armes 1984, Eggermont 1984, Shulman and Goldstein 1984, Tyler, Babin and Niebuhr 1984, Rubin 1984, Gardner 1984).

4

Consulting Specialists

Brian Davis
(West Wales General Hospital, Carmarthen)

The object of this chapter is to follow the likely course of events when an individual seeks medical advice with regard to his or her complaint of tinnitus. The period prior to taking this step may be one of the most unhappy, since many are the dark imaginings that occur when persistent tinnitus first develops. Individual response to tinnitus is, of course, extremely varied and will depend upon other factors that may be present, such as deafness or pain. Certainly, many people will procrastinate when it comes to making that first appointment with their doctor for fear that some awful revelation awaits them. However, clearly this is not in the best interests of the doctor or patient since a delay in diagnosis may mean a delay in treatment. In the particular case of tinnitus the odds are very much in the patient's favour and it is highly probable that following due examination, reassurance that no life-threatening situation exists will be offered.

Additionally in this chapter we shall also take the opportunity to look at some of the possible lines of medical investigation that may be followed. Of course not all investigations will apply to all patients and in this the judgement of the attending family doctor, specialist or consultant is important. Some of the tests will only be necessary when the cause of the tinnitus is far from clear or when further classification or typing of the tinnitus is required to assist in any attempted therapy. Thus, no two patients will necessarily have the same number or types of investigation. What can be said is that none of the tests are of a markedly distressing or painful nature. For the most part they consist of various types of hearing test with the possible addition of X-rays and tests of a small blood sample.

VISITING THE FAMILY DOCTOR

The initial consultation will usually be with the patient's own family doctor who has a sometimes difficult but important screening role in that he must try to decide whether the symptom of tinnitus is due to ear disease or to more generalised bodily disease. Conditions such as anaemia, diabetes mellitus (sugar diabetes), thyroid abnormalities, ototoxicity, high blood pressure, disseminated sclerosis, migraine and meningitis (inflammation of the membranes surrounding the brain), have all been implicated by various authors. Goodey (1981) and Schleuning (1981) consider that infections of head, neck and teeth, abnormalities of the serum lipids (fatty substances carried round in the blood), and autoimmune disease (in which the body's own defence mechanisms mistake part of the body for a foreign material and try to destroy it) should also be considered. Since a wide spectrum of diseases have been related to the production of tinnitus as a symptom, as we noted in a previous chapter, in practice this means that the family doctor will decide whether there is any reason to suspect a generalised disease and, if not, the tinnitus can be provisionally assumed to be due to some form of ear disorder.

One of the first questions, then, to be asked is whether or not the tinnitus has a definite form — that is, is it a meaningful noise such as speech or music? If it is, then it may be a symptom of a psychiatric disorder, it being common, for example, for people with schizophrenia to hear intelligible voices within their head, often giving them messages or instructions. Once it has been established that the sounds are not of the type commonly found in psychiatric illness, then the doctor may enquire as to whether the noise can be heard by people other than the tinnitus sufferer. If those around can also hear the noise of which the individual complains, then it is classified as objective tinnitus, since its presence can be objectively verified by those around. This is a rare form of tinnitus and when it occurs is most often of a 'clicking' nature. The loudness of this is extremely variable, ranging from being audible several feet away from the sufferer to being only just audible through a special form of stethoscope (called a Toynbee tube) inserted into the external canal of the subject's ear.

The vast majority of cases of tinnitus are of the subjective type when only the sufferer can hear the noise. This classical distinction — between subjective and objective forms of tinnitus — has become somewhat blurred in recent times with the use of extremely sensitive microphones placed at the external ear canal. With these it has been

59

possible sometimes to detect spontaneous noise production by the inner part of the ear, which in some cases closely resembles the tinnitus of which the person complains (Kemp 1978). However, for practical purposes the distinction is useful, and objective tinnitus is best regarded as that which can be heard by the examiner without recourse to specialised electronic apparatus. Further points of interest in the patient's history that the doctor will wish to cover include any associated symptoms such as deafness and vertigo, the individual's occupation, past exposure to noise or head injury, family history of deafness and any previous ear problems, including surgery. Before proceeding to examine the ears, a general examination of the patient may be indicated depending upon the history. Certainly the blood pressure should be taken, and especially in a pulsing type of tinnitus it is advisable to listen to the sides of the neck with a stethoscope in case the noise originates in one or other of the great blood vessels in the neck. The family doctor will then proceed to examine the ear using an auriscope, which is a specialised battery-operated instrument that allows for good visual examination of the external ear canal and the ear drum by magnifying and throwing a light onto them. He will have a particular interest in trying to determine whether there is any cause for a conductive deafness. This is a type of deafness due to a defect of the external ear canal, or to the ear drum itself, or of the hammer, anvil and stirrup bones in the middle part of the ear. Conditions such as blockage of the external ear canal by wax, perforation of the ear drum, or collections of pus in the middle part of the ear, may all produce this type of deafness and sometimes associated tinnitus. These conditions may be visually detected by the doctor looking through the auriscope, as, among other things, changes in coloration and shape, and changes in the visual aspect of the middle ear as seen through the ear drum. The use of a tuning fork (one of 512 Hz frequency is most useful, especially if hearing loss is suspected) is to be recommended at this stage since it may be possible to confirm the likely location of the defect and hence by inference the tinnitus and/or hearing loss by using two simple tests. The first of these is the Rinne test in which the subject's hearing is compared between that when a tuning fork is placed with its prongs close alongside the outer ear and that when the base of the tuning fork is pressed firmly on the bony eminence (the mastoid process) behind the ear. A subject with a conductive deafness of 20 dB or more will normally hear the tuning fork most loudly when the base is placed on the mastoid process, and in technical parlance this is termed a negative result or a negative

Rinne. This, however, is not conclusive unless accompanied by the Weber test in which a tuning fork is placed on the top of the skull and the subject asked in which ear the tone is heard most loudly. If a conductive deafness is present in one ear — that is, there is a problem in the conduction of sound from outside the ear to the inner ear — then the tone should be heard loudest in that ear, since there is less competition at the inner ear from external noises. If no conductive loss is present then the tuning fork will merely be heard most loudly in the better of the two ears, or if both ears are equal, it will be heard in the centre of the head.

REFERRAL TO A SPECIALIST

Once the family doctor is fairly satisfied that the tinnitus is due to an otological cause, there is little doubt that the patient should be referred to the Ear, Nose and Throat (ENT) Department of the local hospital for more specialised investigations. Where there is a possible cause from more generalised disease, such as high blood pressure for example, it is reasonable to treat that disease first and then to refer the patient subsequently, should the tinnitus persist. Visiting a specialist on arrival at the ENT Department, the patient's history will once again be taken by the attending specialist. This will broadly follow the outline history already taken by the family doctor, with some increased emphasis on points of particular interest, such as previous exposure to loud noise and drug history. More detailed enquiry will also be made as to the presence of associated symptoms such as vertigo, deafness and discomfort in the ear or ears affected. A formal examination of the ears, nose and throat will then follow. This is a fairly straightforward affair in which the doctor, with the aid of special instruments, examines first the front of the nose, then usually the mouth and the throat, often with the aid of small mirrors that enable him or her to look at the back of the nose and also down at the voice box. Finally the ears will be examined. Depending on the character of the tinnitus the specialist may try to decide whether it is of an objective type by using the Toynbee tube previously mentioned. The specialist will also test the function of the cranial nerves (twelve pairs of nerves that run from the brain to the face and upper part of the body), with particular emphasis on the seventh or facial nerve (which moves the muscles of the face), because it has a close structural, ie. anatomical, relationship with the ear. The corneal reflex may also be tested, which is done by touching a wisp of cotton wool to the cornea of each eye in turn. The patient should blink equally with both eyes at each touch. Delayed or absent blinking on one side only is abnormal. This test detects any significant abnormality in the sensory function of the ophthalmic branch of the trigeminal nerve (the branch of the fifth cranial nerve that runs to the eye). It also tests the motor function of the facial nerve, which supplies the muscles that enable one to blink. The real point of this test is to detect a space-occupying lesion — usually a tumour — that is increasing in size inside the head. Such a tumour on the auditory nerve may interfere with the function of the trigeminal nerve by pressing on it at or near a particular part called the trigeminal ganglion, which lies only a short distance from the auditory nerve within the skull. All in all, this initial examination is useful in that it allows for the detection of any clinically obvious disease such as a tumour at the back of the nose which might, for example, interfere with the functioning of the eustachian tubes and thus cause a conductive deafness with its often associated tinnitus. Or it may detect one or more of the signs of syphillis which might be seen as ulceration in the mouth. Many other conditions may be detected in this way, ranging from thyroid disease to bony abnormalities of the skull, as well as actual middle ear disease. At some stage during the examination the tuning fork tests previously described will also be carried out, after which the examiner will have a good idea of the best lines of investigation that should then be followed in the way of audiometric testing, X-ray and blood analysis.

AUDIOMETRIC TESTING

Pure-tone audiometry

Several types of audiometry — tests of the hearing mechanisms — may be carried out, but it is usual to start with a pure-tone audiogram in which the subject's hearing level for sound between a low pitch of 250 Hz and a high pitch of 8000 Hz is established. For the purposes of this test the subject enters a special sound-proofed room and listens to noises through headphones. A trained audiometric technician carries out the test in which the subject is asked to indicate when he or she can hear the test noises. The method of indicating may range from just raising a hand or nodding, to pressing a button. The sounds will be fed at comfortable levels to the subject via the headphones at intervals between 250 Hz and 8000 Hz until the

Figure 4.1: Audiogram in Menière's syndrome

HEARING LOSS (dB)

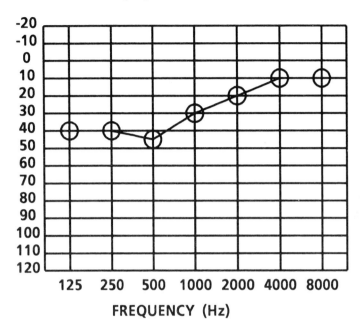

FREQUENCY (Hz)

This figure shows the typical hearing loss associated with Menière's disease. The hearing loss is predominantly in the low-frequency range. A normal audiogram would produce values of around 0 dB hearing loss plus or minus 5 dB at the audiometric frequencies.

audio-metrician has established minimum hearing levels in both ears throughout the frequency range. The result is normally depicted as a graph that shows the amount of hearing loss in decibels at each frequency. Figure 4.1 gives an example.

The shape of this curve is often very important to the examiner. For example, a low-frequency hearing loss associated with a low-frequency tinnitus is compatible with Menière's syndrome, whereas a high-tone hearing loss at 4000 Hz with perhaps some recovery at higher frequencies would be fairly typical of noise-induced hearing loss. Figure 4.2 gives an example.

The hearing loss of old age, known as presbyacusis, tends to produce an audiogram that shows a more and more rapid increase in hearing loss as testing progresses from low to high frequencies.

Figure 4.2: Audiogram in noise-induced hearing loss

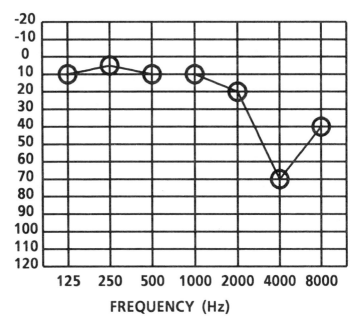

Hearing loss produced as a result of long-term noise exposure usually shows up in the high-frequency region above 4 kHz. The spectral characteristics of the noise will determine the pattern of hearing loss. For example an intense spectral component may produce a 'notch' in the audiogram at a related frequency. However for most types of industrial noise hearing damage is first manifested in hearing loss at high frequencies.

In the full pure-tone audiogram, a form of Rinne test is carried out; hearing for sound fed through the ear canal is compared with that for sound transmitted by a transducer placed over the mastoid process. The minimum hearing thresholds for hearing when sound is conducted by air and when sound is conducted by bone can be compared. Use of this test allows much smaller degrees of conductive deafness to be detected than is possible by using a tuning fork. Furthermore, it is possible to quantify the conductive deafness, which is often helpful, since a very large conductive loss of some 50 to 60 dB, for example, would tend to be associated with an actual

Figure 4.3: Bone and air conduction audiogram showing ossicular discontinuity

HEARING LOSS (dB)

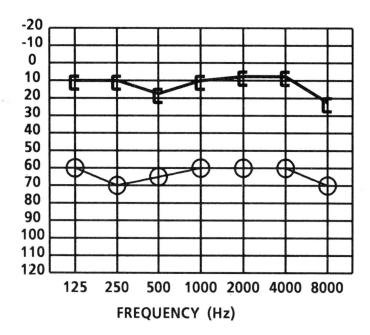

C BONE CONDUCTION

O AIR CONDUCTION

This figure shows a bone-conduction audiogram, where the sound stimulus is applied via a bone vibrator usually to the mastoid process (but sometimes to the frontal bone) and enters the cochlea via vibrations in the surrounding bones. The figure also shows an air conduction audiogram where the sound stimulus is presented to the ear via a headphone. The audiograms show a near-normal bone-conduction audiogram and an air-conduction audiogram that is similar in shape to the bone-conduction audiogram, but which shows about 60 dB hearing loss at all frequencies. The greater hearing loss indicated by the air-conduction audiogram indicates damage to the middle ear, perhaps due to dislocation of the ear ossicles as a consequence of head injury or perhaps to otosclerosis, a bone disease that can result in the stapes becoming fused.

break in the continuity of the bone chain in the middle ear (see figure 4.3 for an example), whereas a much smaller loss of perhaps 20 to 30 dB would be compatible with the presence of fluid in the middle ear.

Where substantial losses are apparent on testing, it is necessary for adequate masking to be used. This is a technique in which wide-band noise — a 'shushing' noise — is fed into the ear not under test while the other ear is being tested. This is necessary especially when testing bone conduction since the skull is a very good conductor of sound, and a sound source placed over one mastoid process produces sound at a level of only 5 or 10 dB less in the opposite ear. Thus it is possible, when a subject has severe conductive deafness on one side, for him or her to think, when the sound is placed on the mastoid process of that side, that it is being heard in that ear, whereas in reality it is being heard in the other ear. By feeding wide-band noise of sufficient volume into the good ear, it is possible to fully occupy that ear (by the masking noise) so that it does not detect noise conducted from the other side of the skull, thus allowing testing of one ear at a time. Any significant conductive deafness may be due to such factors as otosclerosis, in which superfluous bone forms on the bones of the middle ear thus reducing their ability to transmit vibrations, or secretory otitis media (glue ear), both of which are treatable conditions, although the tinnitus associated with otosclerosis is not necessarily relieved by an operation that restores the hearing.

Impedance audiometry

If a conductive deafness has been found, then impedance audiometry may be carried out. This is essentially a technique to measure middle ear pressure and the ease of movement (the compliance) of the ear drum and bone chain in the middle ear. It is a painless investigation carried out by inserting a probe, which has three channels, into the ear under investigation. The first channel is used to emit sound and the second channel to receive sound; the third channel is used to vary the pressure in the external ear canal. The probe has to fit tightly enough to provide an air-tight seal in order that the pressure may be varied. Sounds are absorbed by the ear drum most efficiently when the pressure on either side of it is equal. Therefore the external pressure at which the least amount of sound is returned to the probe is that which equals the pressure in the middle ear.

Figure 4.4: Tympanogram showing normal and reduced middle ear pressure

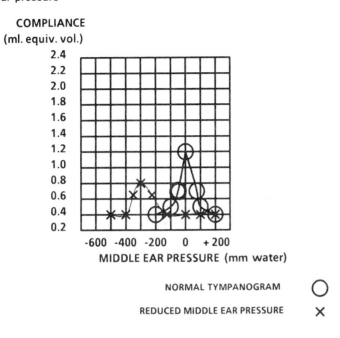

COMPLIANCE
(ml. equiv. vol.)

MIDDLE EAR PRESSURE (mm water)

NORMAL TYMPANOGRAM O

REDUCED MIDDLE EAR PRESSURE X

The compliance of the ear is measured by determining the reflection of a low-frequency probe-tone in a sealed auditory canal while the air-pressure in the canal is varied (see text). The compliance is greatest when the air-pressure in the canal is equal to that in the middle ear. The figure shows both a normal tympanogram and also one that indicates reduced middle-ear pressure, which may be the result of a blockage in the eustachian tube.

Subjects with eustachian tube disorders generally have a relatively low middle ear pressure revealed by this test. Figure 4.4 gives an example of this.

The shape of the curve traced by the machine during the variation in pressure may be helpful in diagnosis (Jerger 1970, Feldman 1975). For example, a completely flat curve indicates a middle ear full of fluid, which is, of course, relatively incompressible, and therefore allows little movement of the ear drum.

An unusually high compliance — i.e. a lot of ear drum movement — may indicate some form of discontinuity of the ossicular bone chain. Figure 4.5 gives an illustration.

Figure 4.5: Tympanogram: flat curve showing otitis media and high curve showing ossicular discontinuity

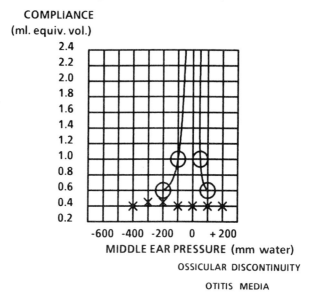

This figure shows the tympanogram characteristic of otitis media, which produces a flat curve because the middle ear in this condition is full of fluid instead of air, and a high curve showing increased compliance indicating ossicular discontinuity or alternatively ear drum abnormality.

The stapedial reflex

It is customary when carrying out impedance audiometry not only to measure the middle ear pressure and the compliance of the ear drum, but also to examine a specialised response known as the stapedial reflex. This reflex is a response to loud noise of the order of 80 dB or more, in which there is automatic tensing of an extremely small muscle that attaches to the stapes bone in the middle ear, which conveys vibration to the inner ear. It is thought to be a protection against extremely loud noise because when the muscle tenses it partially fixes the stapes and so reduces sound conduction to the inner ear. By feeding loud sound into the ear at 80 dB or above during the impedance test, it is possible to bring the reflex into play, in which case it reduces the sound conduction by the middle ear bones and consequently there is an increase in sound reflected back from the ear drum to the probe. Thus the sound level at which this sudden increase in reflected sound is detected is the intensity required to produce the stapedial reflex in a particular individual. This test is one of the few objective tests of a part of the hearing mechanism (that is, it is a test in which the mechanism is assessed without the need for the subject's verbal report).

The stapedial reflex may be absent when there is fixation of the stapes by diseases such as otosclerosis or when deafness is sufficiently severe to make it impossible to obtain high enough noise levels to initiate the reflex. The stapedial reflex is what is called a crossed reflex, in that noise fed into one ear initiates reflex in *both* ears and so provides a method of testing not only sound reception by the ear receiving the noise, but also the motor function of the facial nerve that supplies the little stapedius muscle on the opposite or on the same side. This may be important when tumours of the auditory nerve are suspected, since they can interfere with the function of the facial nerve. In fact, this aspect of the test has been much refined and measurements of decay and latency of the reflex may be carried out. For measurement of decay, the persistence of the reflex in the presence of a prolonged eliciting sound is measured. Typically, the noise stimulus is presented for ten seconds at 1000 Hz at a level just sufficient to bring about the reflex — as found by previous testing. The continuation of the reflex — i.e. the continued tensing of the small muscle connected to the stapes — is then observed by monitoring the amount of sound being reflected back from the ear drum. If this falls to less than 50 per cent of its original value within a ten-second period, then abnormal reflex delay is said to be present. This quite strongly suggests auditory nerve damage or tumour in the region of the connection of the auditory nerve with the brain itself (Anderson, Barr and Wedenberg 1969). The reflex latency is really a measure of the reflex delay or the time it takes to start. Once again the stapedial reflex is initiated with a suitable noise and the interval between starting the noise and the appearance of the stapedial reflex is measured. Abnormal prolongation of this interval is again very suggestive of damage to the auditory nerve or its connections to the brain.

Recruitment

Finally, with regard to stapedial reflex testing, mention must be made of recruitment, which is a phenomenon characterised by deafness at low noise intensities but normal hearing at higher noise intensities. It is very characteristic of deafness due to damage in the inner ear. Thus, a person with quite severe but recruiting deafness

Figure 4.6 Loudness balance test to differentiate a recruiting deafness

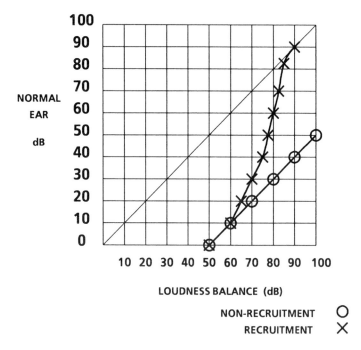

LOUDNESS BALANCE (dB)

NON-RECRUITMENT   O

RECRUITMENT   X

This figure shows the results of a Fowler's loudness balance test for unilateral recruiting deafness and for unilateral non-recruiting deafness. Note that for the recruiting deafness, tones at high sound levels (above 80 dB SPL) produce the same loudness in both the normal and deaf ear.

may have a stapedial reflex that occurs at or near the normal relatively loud (80 dB) sound level. This in itself is an additional diagnostic aid that helps the examiner to distinguish between deafness due to inner ear damage with recruitment, or to auditory nerve damage without recruitment. The presence of recruitment can be confirmed when there is a symmetric hearing loss by an investigation known as Fowler's loudness balance test. Here the subject is asked to balance identical sounds, usually tones, of different intensities in each ear. At low sound intensities the ear with recruiting deafness will require a higher sound intensity than the normal ear for the subject to say the two sounds are in balance. But, as the overall intensity is increased, the difference in sound level required for balance will gradually disappear since at higher sound levels the recruiting ear will start to hear as well as the normal ear. Figure 4.6 gives an example of this.

A less accurate test of recruitment is that of loudness discomfort levels in which a patient is exposed to sound of increasing intensity until discomfort is complained of. If this is at normal or near-normal levels of discomfort, then the patient can be assumed to have a recruiting deafness.

Bekesy and speech audiometry

Other tests that help the clinician distinguish between problems due to inner ear disease and problems due to auditory nerve damage include tone decay and speech and Bekesy audiometry. The test for tone decay examines the patient's ability to hear a continuous tone a little above his or her hearing threshold. Patients with damage of the auditory nerve have great difficulty hearing a continuous tone of low intensity for more than a very short period of time, whereas those with a normal auditory nerve have little difficulty. During the test the intensity of the tone is steadily increased if the patient is unable to keep hearing it, until it is continuously heard for one minute. The size of the increase above the subject's hearing threshold needed to hear the tone for one minute is termed the tone decay, and is usually in excess of 30 dB in individuals with auditory nerve damage. Bekesy audiometry is a routine investigation in many ENT Departments although increasingly it has been replaced by other test procedures such as those already described. The Bekesy audiometer traces a curve as a result of the subject's responses first of all to a continuous and then to an interrupted pure tone. This is usually achieved by the subject pressing a button whenever the noise is audible. As long as the button is pressed the intensity of the noise easily reduces. When the noise can no longer be heard, the subject releases the button, whereupon the intensity steadily increases. All the while, independent of the button pressing, the noise is gradually sweeping through the frequencies from low to high. In this way a somewhat saw-toothed hearing threshold curve is obtained for each ear for both continuous and for interrupted tones. The degree and manner of overlap of the continuous and interrupted hearing threshold for each ear may provide useful inferential information with regard to the site of origin of the hearing problem and tinnitus. Figure 4.7 gives an example.

Figure 4.7: Bekesy audiogram for normal hearing and for cochlear damage

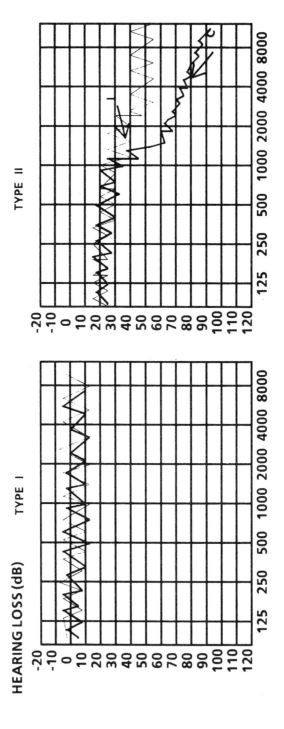

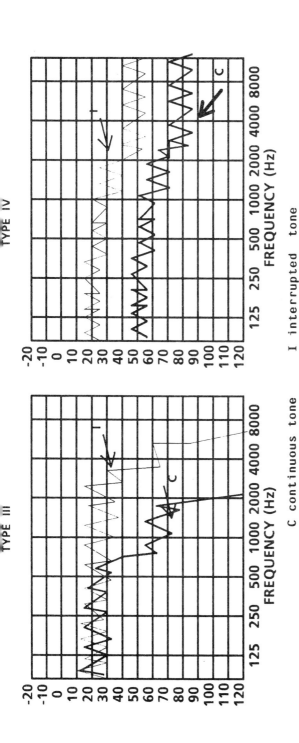

The figure shows Jerger's (1960) classification of Bekesy audiograms for continuous (C) and interrupted (I) tones (see text). Type I, where there is an interweaving of the continuous and interrupted tones indicates normal hearing. Type II, where the continuous trace becomes separated from the interrupted trace and where the oscillations in the continuous trace become smaller, indicates loudness recruitment and is characteristic of a cochlear site of hearing damage. Type III is prevalent in a retrocochlear pathology. Type IV, where there is an early separation of the continuous and interrupted traces would also be indicative of retrocochlear lesion.

Figure 4.8: Speech audiogram showing normal hearing, cochlear deafness and nerve deafness

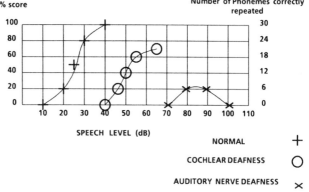

The speech audiogram is a plot of recognition score for short words or phonemes against the intensity of the speech signal. The plot for normal hearing is sigmoid in shape. A similar shape is seen for conductive deafness but the curve is shifted towards higher speech levels. Auditory nerve or sensorineural deafness, when there is recruitment, produces a different shape (a parabola), which shows that after a certain level recognition performance deteriorates.

Speech audiometry is another routine test that may give useful information in sensorineural deafness when trying to decide whether the defect responsible lies in the inner ear or in the auditory nerve. It has been observed that subjects with auditory nerve damage have much poorer speech comprehension than those with cochlear damage only, although their pure-tone audiogram may be quite satisfactory. Thus, in speech audiometry, a pure-tone audiogram is first obtained and then the individual's response to speech at different intensities of sound is monitored and compared with the pure-tone audiogram to see whether the former is disproportionately low. The test is usually conducted by the subject being asked to listen to lists of monosyllabic words, such as get, met, not, and so on, often arranged in groups of ten, while the examiner varies the sound intensity. The sound level at which half the words are consistently correctly understood is designated the speech reception threshold and should normally be within 30 dB of the average pure-tone threshold over the speech frequency range. However, the test is usually conducted in a slightly more sophisticated manner in that the subject's percentage correct score is plotted at various noise intensities from 0 to 100 decibels. An S-shaped (sigmoid) curve is plotted for the normal ear, with 100 per cent discrimination being reached at around the 40 dB level. With damage to the auditory nerve it may be impossible for the subject to score more than 30 per cent, even at high volumes, although the pure-tone audiogram may have shown little or no hearing loss. Figure 4.8 gives an example of this.

Tests of the organ of balance

A patient who has been through all or most of the previously described tests may consider himself to have been well investigated for all normal purposes. However, a test for balance (vestibular function) may sometimes be indicated, since the organs of balance are closely related to the hearing mechanism in the inner ear. This is the one test that may occasion the subject a small amount of discomfort in that at some stage the sensation of spinning with the possible addition of mild nausea will be induced. This is quite normal, quickly passes, and need cause no alarm. The test itself is carried out by putting water or air that has been cooled or warmed 7°C below or above body temperature into the external ear canals — referred to as irrigating the ears. During this irrigation, which normally lasts for 30 seconds, the movements of the eye are monitored by small electrodes placed on the forehead. These detect changes in electrical activity with eye movement. Normally a flicking movement of the eye from side to side, termed a nystagmus, is induced. Closer inspection of this reveals that the flicking movement is more rapid in one direction than the other. Such a nystagmus is described as having a fast and a slow phase. By convention it is named after the fast phase. Thus, if the eye repeatedly moves slowly to the right and then flicks quickly back to the left, it would be described as a nystagmus to the left. Warm irrigation of an ear produces a nystagmus towards that ear. Cold irrigation produces a nystagmus away from that ear. By irrigating each ear, it is possible to compare the responses on each side to see how much out of balance they may be. The point of particular interest is the speed of the slow phase of the nystagmus. This may be markedly reduced in one ear, in which case a defect of that balance organ is identified, and is normally referred to as a paresis (weakness) of that labyrinth. This test is considered to be important in instances in which there is a need to confirm the diagnosis of Menière's syndrome or there is a need to investigate further the possibility of an acoustic neuroma, since such a tumour may indirectly affect the performance of the balance organ by pressure on the vestibular nerve. Additionally there is a school of thought that considers that some forms of tinnitus may be due to primary pathology of the vestibular system itself (Shulman 1984).

TINNITUS CLINICS

Should the individual attend a specialised centre or tinnitus clinic, it is possible that further diagnostic tests may be employed, but these are essentially of a research nature and are not routinely used unless there is some specific identifiable problem that cannot be resolved by other means. The mainstay of these tests is the averaging computer, which allows consistent reproducible electrical physiological responses of the auditory system to be separated from a mass of other physiological activity. This necessitates a series of readings being taken and fed into the computer, which then allows any consistent waveform to emerge. The simplest test of this nature is the post-auricular myogenic response, in which an electrode is placed over the small muscles just beneath the skin behind the ear. In lower mammals these muscles move the ears in response to sound and, although somewhat vestigial in humans, they still have a detectable electrical response to sound in most people. The measurement of this muscle response to sound provides an objective test of hearing, often to within 30 dB of actual hearing threshold. Since the response is absent in many adults, this is in no way a conclusive screening test, and most centres prefer to concentrate on a combination of electrocochleography and brain-stem evoked response audiometry. Electrocochleography requires that a needle electrode should be placed through the ear drum to touch the inner wall of the middle ear. This may be done with local or general anaesthetic. Other electrodes are placed behind the ear and on the skull, and a series of 'clicking' noises are fed into the ear under test. The electrical responses of the ear and auditory nerve are recorded by the averaging computer. The clinically most useful of the electrical response characteristics is the conduction wave (action potential) of the auditory nerve. Not only does monitoring this allow the estimation of a fairly accurate objective hearing threshold, but the form of the wave itself may assist diagnosis of conditions such as acoustic neuroma or Menière's Disease. Brain-stem electrical response audiometry is a technique

Figure 4.9: Brainstem electrical response (evoked onset brainstem potentials to click stimulus (schematic representation))

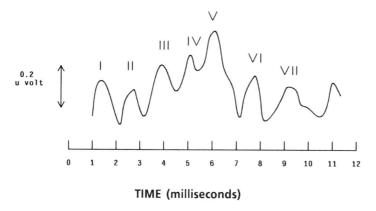

TIME (milliseconds)

This figure shows a schematic representation of the averaged brain-stem electrical response to a brief sound stimulus (see text). The two most stable peaks are thought to indicate neural activity produced by processing of the sound stimulus in the primary cochlear nuclei (wave II) and the inferior colliculus (wave V).

somewhat similar to the electrocochleography in that it requires the use of the averaging computer and a large number of repetitive sound stimuli. But in this case only surface electrodes are used, being normally placed on the forehead and over the mastoid processes. Using this technique it is possible to monitor the electrical activity from the auditory nerve through various pathways to the brain itself. In practice seven distinct waves are identified, of which the fifth wave is considered the most clinically useful. Figure 4.9 shows an example of the waveform.

The interval between the sound stimulus and the fifth wave can be measured and if prolonged is an indicator of an acoustic neuroma. Large acoustic neuromas may cause a complete loss of all waves apart from the first. Although the various audiological and vestibular function tests provide the mainstay of diagnosis in patients with tinnitus, X-ray (radiology) and blood test investigations are frequently necessary additions, either as part of the investigation for more generalised disease, or, especially in the case of radiology, for further investigation of specific ear disease. When there is reason to suspect disease involving the mastoid bone or the middle ear, X-ray of the mastoid bones may be requested. If there is any suspicion of

77

acoustic neuroma, the X-ray of the internal auditory meatus (the bony canals through which the auditory nerves run) may be requested, since widening of these canals is indicative of damage. More rarely, a specialised X-ray known as a tomograph may be indicated, which, especially when computer-assisted, can give a startlingly clear picture of the internal anatomy of the skull and ears. However, this is an expensive technique and also requires an increased exposure to X-rays, so it is not used as a matter of routine. It must be emphasised that none of the radiological examinations described should cause any distress to the subject whatsoever, since they are entirely painless and are usually conducted in a friendly and pleasant atmosphere. Investigations of the blood generally have a low priority in the investigation of tinnitus but it is generally considered wise to test for syphilis, although this is a very rare cause nowadays. It is important that the FTA (fluorescent treponemal antibody) absorption test be requested, otherwise cases of syphilis may be missed. Additionally, the patient should be tested for anaemia, and, especially in cases of acute onset deafness in the younger age groups, a serum lipid profile should be ordered.

In a tinnitus clinic an attempt will be made to match the tinnitus sound to an external machine-produced sound, so that its characteristics can be described and examined for both research and masking therapy purposes. Various types and levels of masking sound will be introduced for the individual to listen to, and these more specialised aspects of the investigation are considered in the next chapters. Of necessity it has been possible in this chapter to give only an outline of the medical techniques that may be employed in the specialised investigation of the person with tinnitus. However, it is hoped that sufficient information has been given to enable an intelligent understanding of most of the procedures and to allay any anxieties with regard to the discomfort or safety of the investigations.

5

Tinnitus Assessment

To date there is not a universally accepted classification of tinnitus. This perhaps reflects the fact that in many cases the actual mechanism responsible for producing tinnitus is unknown and also it can be difficlt to determine whether the site of production of the tinnitus is of peripheral (the cochlea or auditory nerve) or of central origin (auditory cortex). Part of the problem of tinnitus is that it is extremely difficult to assess accurately and the aim of this chapter is to explain how an assessment and a 'characterisation' or typing of an individual's tinnitus can be obtained.

The assessment of tinnitus would generally require prior testing of the hearing ability of both ears. These tests have been described in Chapter 4 and basically would include the following: obtaining the audiogram to ascertain the degree of hearing loss at selected frequencies, tests for recruitment, impedance audiometry and tests to determine the presence of conductive or sensorineural deafness. These tests and other psychophysical tests, together with self-reports by the tinnitus subject, enable a profile of the tinnitus to be built up. The profile would include a number of personal details such as the age and sex of the sufferer, as well as the age at onset of the tinnitus and a verbal description of the tinnitus at present and any information regarding the way the tinnitus may have changed in nature since it was first noticed. The following psychophysical tests can be used to obtain a more precise description of the tinnitus.

LATERALISATION OF TINNITUS

Consideration of the subject's report of the site of tinnitus is an important step in the characterisation of an individual's tinnitus, since a number of other tests depend upon this knowledge. The tinnitus may be reported by the subject as being only in one ear. This is termed *unilateral tinnitus*. If the hearing is near normal in the other, non-tinnitus, ear then comparison stimuli can be applied to the non-tinnitus ear. Often the subject reports that tinnitus is present at both ears, and this is termed *bilateral tinnitus*. The tinnitus may be of a similar nature in both ears or it may be quite distinguishable in character. In the case of bilateral tinnitus the assessment may proceed independently for both ears, although preferably in different testing sessions. The subject may also report the tinnitus as being within the head and lateralised to one side or the other.

Tinnitus, in nearly all cases, is heard as lateralised rather than localised.[1] Although the subject may report the tinnitus as being within the head this does not necessarily imply a central site for the tinnitus (McFadden 1982). If there are similar types of tinnitus at the two ears, then the tinnitus may be heard as within the head, either at the middle of the head, if the two tinnitus signals are of a similar loudness or strength, or towards the side of the louder tinnitus. Sometimes this can be demonstrated by masking the tinnitus at one ear so that the tinnitus in the other ear is clearly heard at the side opposite to the masking stimulus. If this does not occur then it is possible that the tinnitus is centrally sited, which may indicate a neural lesion as the site of the tinnitus. There is some evidence that two similar tinnitus signals at the two ears do not merge into a 'central lateralised tinnitus', as would in general be the case with external sounds, but rather remain as distinct sensations located at the ears (Vernon 1978).

LOUDNESS TEST

In order to obtain some idea of the loudness of the tinnitus it is usual to adjust the intensity of a comparison sound (usually a tone at 1 kHz) until the subject reports that the comparison sound is similar in loudness to the tinnitus. The value used to characterise the loudness of the tinnitus is then either the sensation level in dB of the comparison tone (i.e. the difference between the hearing threshold of the comparison tone and the dB SPL level at which it matches the tinnitus in loudness), or the dBA level of the comparison tone. In general, the dBA level is to be preferred because of the problem of recruitment (Goodwin and Johnstone 1980; Tyler and Conrad-Armes 1983). The problem with using the dB SPL measure is that if the comparison tone is situated within an area of hearing loss, and in a situation where recruitment is present, then the tone rapidly grows in loudness as it is increased in intensity above the hearing threshold. Therefore, when loudness recruitment is present, a sound that is only a few dB above hearing threshold may sound as loud as that same tone which is presented to a normal ear. Hence, if the tinnitus is quoted in dB sensation level, then there may be a serious under-estimation of the perceived loudness of the tinnitus.

There are, however, many problems in attaining a confident reliable estimate of the loudness of tinnitus. First, the comparison tone may itself have a masking effect on the tinnitus, or the tone may produce residual inhibition of the tinnitus (see below). This is particularly the case if the comparison tone cannot be presented to the opposite ear from the tinnitus, for instance when the subject is completely deaf in the non-tinnitus ear. The tinnitus sufferer may also object that the tinnitus does not sound like the comparison tone. Whatever the result of a loudness test, it has to be remembered that even a quiet sound can be extremely annoying and that a low loudness match should not be taken to indicate that the tinnitus itself is insignificant.

TINNITUS ANNOYANCE

To quantify this aspect of tinnitus is difficult. Annoyance is not simply a function of loudness or complexity. In a recent study, (Terry and Jones 1986) tinnitus sufferers as well as normal-hearing subjects related, in terms of annoyance, a variety of sounds that comprised both sounds which could be used as tinnitus maskers and other sounds of varying degrees of annoyance. The tinnitus sufferers and the normal-hearing subjects rated the sounds in a broadly similar fashion.

The tinnitus sufferer, however, may judge his own tinnitus to be highly annoying. The fact that the sufferer has no control over the tinnitus is likely to be a major factor in annoyance rather than the loudness or nature of the tinnitus. This may be one of the reasons why a tinnitus-masking noise is often preferred to the tinnitus itself and this point is discussed further in Chapter 15.

PITCH MATCH

It is often the case that the tinnitus is of a tonal type (a narrow band spectral component) and has a definite pitch. Other non-tonal types also can have a pitch-like quality and it is useful to attempt to obtain a pitch match. Again it is preferable to present the comparison tone to the opposite ear from the tinnitus and also to give the subject control over the intensity of the tone, so as to keep the loudness of the comparison tone and tinnitus match of similar value. The subject should also be able to switch off the tone (or to have the tone pulsed on and off), to aid comparison between the tone and the tinnitus. Pitch matching of high-frequency tones can be quite difficult, particularly if the sensitivity of the two ears differ, and for mid-frequency tones there is the possibility of octave confusions. The pitch match should therefore be repeated several times to improve and check the reliability of the measure.

Preferably the subject should also try to match two objective tones in pitch to determine whether the individual can indeed make such a match. It is of interest that it has been recently reported that while subjects may make accurate pitch matches of two external tones they do not, in general, make consistent pitch matches to their tinnitus (Penner 1981). This may indicate that tonal tinnitus varies substantially between and even within a testing session. Alternatively, such a finding is in accord with the view that tinnitus cannot be treated as a special case of an external tone or noise.

The pitch match, nevertheless, may prove useful in determining the cause of tinnitus. For example, a reasonably high pitch match above 2 kHz may be sufficient to rule out Menière's Disease, since a low roar or rumble is generally associated with this cause of tinnitus (Douek and Reid 1968).

SYNTHESIS MATCH

The availability of reasonably inexpensive synthesisers has led to efforts to obtain a synthesised match to tinnitus (Hazell 1980). In the cases in which the tinnitus is a complex sound, then attempts to obtain a simple pitch match with a pure tone may prove frustrating and not particularly informative. The synthesiser allows an almost unlimited variety of sounds to be used in attempting to find a match with the tinnitus. However, obtaining a reasonable match to a complex tinnitus can be a long process, possibly a matter of hours, even with an experienced operator of the synthesiser. It also has to be kept in mind that the tinnitus itself may vary over this period and so several matches over several sessions would be required before confidence could be placed in a synthesised match to a complex tinnitus. Nevertheless, a finer class of categorisation of tinnitus types may be possible with this technique and study of this data could be informative to the clinician.

TINNITUS-MASKED AUDIOGRAM

The masked audiogram, in relation to tinnitus assessment, is made by determining the minimum intensity of a tone or a band of noise at which the tinnitus is just masked (that is the tinnitus cannot be heard above the tone or the noise masker). This determination is made for different frequencies of the tone (or centre frequencies of the band of noise). The frequencies chosen are usually the same as the audiometric frequencies used in determining hearing sensitivity, although it is often useful to include additional frequencies to improve resolution. (It may be useful at this point to encourage the movement of the upper limit of audiometric measurement from 8 kHz to at least 12 kHz, since there has been a general improvement of equipment and headphones, and change in hearing sensitivity at high frequencies may give early warning of more serious damage to the mid-frequency range.) Figure 5.1 gives some examples of the types of masked audiograms that can be obtained. Work by Feldmann (1971, 1983) has been particularly useful in setting up a typology of tinnitus based on the comparison of the normal and masked audiograms.

To explain this figure, let us for the moment treat the tinnitus as an external tone. If the frequency of the tone was 2 kHz and its level 30 dB HL (dB above the hearing threshold), then the masking audiogram (or maskgram) would show that as masking tones move in frequency away from 2 kHz (say to 125 Hz and 4 kHz), the tones have to be increasingly intense in order to mask the 2 kHz tone. However, for tones close to 2 kHz, the tones do not have to be as intense for the 2 kHz tone to be masked. The shape of the curve therefore tells something about the position of the 2 kHz tone, and if we were to repeat the procedure for another tone of unknown frequency then the frequency region of the tone could be deduced from the maskgram. Although tinnitus does not in general behave as an external tone, determining a maskgram for the tinnitus can often

Figure 5.1: The masked audiogram as a tool for providing a typology of tinnitus

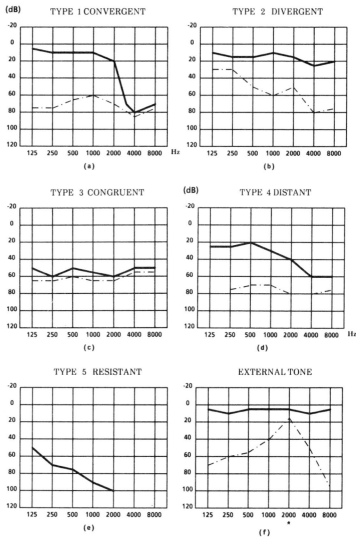

In each of the graphs the solid line represents the threshold audiogram, while the dashed line represents the level of a tone in dB above the normal hearing threshold required to mask the tinnitus. In (e) it is not possible to mask the tinnitus (resistant type). In (f) a masked audiogram for an external tone of 2 kHz is shown. The curves shown are idealised examples to show the different types of masked audiogram. (Adapted from Feldmann 1971, Figure 1.)

prove useful in terms of classification. However, it should be emphasised that poor frequency resolution, as would be expected in cases of cochlear and nerve disorder, would produce a broader masking curve, even though the tinnitus was localised in one region. Thus, interpretation of the tinnitus masking curve would also require information on the frequency resolution of the auditory system of the tinnitus sufferer (Tyler *et al.* 1980, Shailer *et al.* 1980).

Feldmann's classification was into five basic types and these are described below together with the percentage of tinnitus cases of each type found in the 1971 study:

1. Convergence: This is when the threshold (normal audiogram) and the masking curves (maskgram) converge towards the higher frequencies. This type of tinnitus is usually of high pitch and there is associated high-frequency hearing loss. Often the cause of the hearing loss is long-term exposure to industrial noise. About 34 per cent of cases were of this type.

2. Divergence: In this type the threshold and masking curves diverge from low to high frequencies. The tinnitus pitch in this case would be low. However this type is much rarer than the convergent type, with only 3 per cent of cases being classified as 'divergent type'.

3. Congruence: This is when the audiogram and maskgram coincide. This type is often associated with Menière's Disease and otosclerosis. Thirty-two per cent of cases examined were classified as 'congruent type'.

4. Distant: This is when the audiogram and maskgram are separated at all points by 10 dB or more, which would indicate that the masker would be perceived as moderately loud. About 20 per cent of cases were classified as distant type.

5. Resistant: This is when the tinnitus can not be masked by tones or noise at any intensity level. This type is found in cases of severe sensorineural hearing loss, when the amount of activation of the auditory system by even an intense masker noise would be small, so that the sensation due to the masker would not be sufficient to 'swamp' the tinnitus. However, it is possible to find cases in which an intense masker is perceived as loud but yet the tinnitus is still heard (Vernon and Meikle 1981).

It is important in these cases to establish whether binaurally presented maskers can mask the tinnitus, since in the case of bilateral tinnitus, the subject may fail to report a change in the lateralisation of the tinnitus when masking is only applied to one ear. Feldmann does not give a figure for the percentage of cases of the 'resistant type' but a figure of about 10 per cent is implied.

If the tinnitus could be treated as an external tonal stimulus then the shape of the maskgram would be like a tone-on-tone masking curve (Wegel and Lane 1924). Feldmann did not see cases of this type and concludes that tinnitus does not in general behave like an external tone. If the tinnitus were to behave like an external tone then one might see a tinnitus maskgram resembling an inverted 'V' shape, when the tinnitus was of medium pitch and when little or no hearing loss was present. In this type the audiogram may have a notch at a similar frequency position as the peak position of the maskgram.

RESIDUAL INHIBITION

This term refers to the phenomenon when tinnitus is suppressed either completely or partially following exposure to a masking stimulus. The effect was apparently first noted by A.J. Spaulding, an otolaryngologist who, when playing his violin to tinnitus patients in an attempt to match tinnitus pitch, noticed that a sustained note could sometimes reduce or suppress the tinnitus (Vernon 1981). In subjects in whom residual inhibition (RI) is easily induced the subject may spontaneously report a decrease or drop in the level of the tinnitus when the maskgram is being determined. However, the demonstration of RI may critically depend on the nature of the masker. A simple test for RI would be to present a masking sound, a tone or wide-band noise, at a level at least 10 dB SPL above the level at which the tinnitus was masked, for a duration of one minute. The subject is then asked to report any changes in the loudness of the tinnitus when the masker is turned off, as compared with the loudness level of the tinnitus before the masker was presented. Another method would be to use a continuous loudness balance to measure the time-course of the RI (Terry, Jones, Davis & Slater 1983). When the masker is turned off, there is often a dramatic decrease in the tinnitus loudness level, with the tinnitus gradually returning to its original loudness. Although in other cases no loudness reduction occurs and sometimes tinnitus loudness increases.

A significant amount of RI is obviously of importance in terms of treatment of the tinnitus. It would also be of clinical value if the nature of the RI response could be used to differentiate tinnitus types or provide information on the site of lesion producing the tinnitus.

However it has proved difficult to establish any such correlation, although a recent large-scale investigation into the effectiveness of tinnitus masking may provide an answer to this question (Hazell *et al.* 1985).

In this study a laboratory test of residual inhibition or enhancement (i.e. if the masking sound led subsequently to an increase in loudness of the tinnitus) was given to groups of tinnitus sufferers partaking in a trial of tinnitus maskers. The test given was to use a wide-band noise (WBN) as a masker and to present this, for a period of one minute, at 10 dB above the level at which tinnitus was just masked (or at 5 dB below any at which the subject shows any sign of discomfort or at 130 dB SPL — whichever is the lowest level). The subject was asked to note the level of the tinnitus before the presentation of the masker and to compare that with the level immediately after the masker was turned off. The subject reported whether the tinnitus was softer or louder than before the presentation of the masker or whether the tinnitus had disappeared. The experimenter also noted the time it took for the subject to report that the tinnitus had returned to the original level (exact details of the test are given in Hazell *et al.* 1985). It appeared that presence of RI was evenly distributed throughout different age groups and also evenly distributed with relation to the different tinnitus pitches recorded in this sample. The conclusion from this study would be that the presence of RI is evenly distributed between tinnitus types.

The results of the above tests and the previous medical tests should serve to categorise the tinnitus and may well be sufficient to identify the cause and site of tinnitus and to suggest possible treatment. However, in other cases the site and cause of the tinnitus may still remain unknown.

NOTES

1. The term localisation is strictly to be kept for sounds that are heard as being located in the external auditory space — lateralisation is the term referring to sounds that are reported as being at the ears or within the head. Normal stereophonic recordings played over headphones give the effect of sounds or music heard within the head. If, however, the recordings are made with microphones placed in dummy heads (so that the transformation due to the effect of the artificial pinna and head is present in the sound recorded by the microphone) then, when listening to the recordings with headphones, there is a sensation of the sounds as being localised in auditory space.

6

The Incidence of Tinnitus

Tinnitus must have existed for as long as people have walked the earth — and probably existed before *Homo sapiens*, the species label that we give to ourselves. Why? Because tinnitus in many instances is symptomatic of a malfunction of the auditory system, be it in the outer, middle or inner ear, in the nerve pathways from the ear to the brain, or in that area of the brain — the auditory cortex — that processes the signals from the ears. If faults in this highly complex system can give rise to tinnitus in modern man there is every reason to believe the problem existed for primitive man. However, the extent of the problem may have been greater in more recent times since we know tinnitus is linked to noise exposure (Coles, Davies and Haggard 1981). The auditory system evolved to detect fairly low intensity sounds in a more-or-less quiet background — to detect enemies stalking around in the bush, so to speak — which is hardly the state of affairs in our hearing environment today.

Perhaps the most recent aspect of environmental noise to give cause for concern is that concerning pop music: pop concerts, discos and personal stereos. Of the last it is clear from a study by Grover (1984) that while personal cassette recorders can give output levels high enough to be harmful with prolonged use, typical listening levels fall into a grey area in this respect. He urges that an alarmist view is not taken but that users should not turn up the volume any higher than there is any real need to. One risk, of course, is that since the players can be worn in environments that are themselves noisy (e.g. while cycling in traffic) the chances are that they will often be played at volumes higher than would be needed in one's own front room. Little is yet known about the extent of use of these cassette players but until further research is undertaken one must accept that they may present a potential risk to the frequent user (Miller and Jakimetz 1984).

PROBLEMS WITH QUESTIONS

As we shall see, there is some — perhaps inescapable — controversy surrounding the prevalence figures for tinnitus. The reason for this is straightforward although the rectification of the problem behind it is less so. At present there are no strictly objective measures of the existence of tinnitus in most people who report it. There is as yet no 'machine' that can be fixed directly to someone's head that can produce irrefutable evidence that the person has tinnitus. Until such a day arrives, the evidence available is that provided by the individual him or herself — it depends on his or her verbal report.

Incidence statistics are produced from various forms of sample surveys, where a sub-sample of the entire population is chosen, often in such a way that the figures arising from a survey of the sub-sample can be generalised with a known degree of accuracy to the population at large. Unless a census is done of the entire population in which everyone is asked the question, the available figures at best can only give a range within which the population figure is likely to lie, given an acceptable degree of certainty. Sampling statistics enable one to say 'I am 99 per cent sure' — i.e. I may be wrong on one occasion in a 100 — 'that the number of people with tinnitus in the population lies between x per cent and y per cent'. Few surveys into tinnitus have attained such a degree of statistical sophistication, and those that have, although confident in the generality of their results, refrain from explicitly stating what the 'certainty' level is, and what the *range* of the estimate for the population is.

That apart, the major problem remains, namely that verbal reports depend on the questions that elicit them, and designing the ultimate set of 'foolproof' questions to elicit meaningful figures on the incidence of tinnitus is no easy task. Most people would probably say that at some time or other they have experienced something akin to 'ringing in the ears'. Indeed, most people may actually be able to hear head noises, given the appropriate sound-proofed environment. For example, Heller and Bergman (1953), in an often-cited (but apparently unrepeated) study, placed 80 people, who said they had normal hearing and no evidence of aural disease, into a sound-proof chamber and asked them to make notes of any sounds that they could hear. Over 90 per cent noted one or two noises that they described in similar terms — as buzzing, humming, ringing, etc. This is a small sample to generalise from, and there may be an element of suggestion at work, in that asking subjects to make notes of anything they heard might have implied they would hear something.

As yet no schedule of questions has been universally agreed upon as a standard protocol for prevalence surveys of tinnitus. Clearly, the way questions are worded, particularly when an attempt is made to gauge the severity of the tinnitus in a survey, can influence the eventual incidence figures and it is likely that differences in question phrasing explain some of the differences in incidence figures from different surveys (Coles 1984a).

AMERICAN INCIDENCE FIGURES

The American National Health survey estimated in 1968 that 36 million American adults (approximately 20 per cent of the population) suffered from tinnitus, which was 'severe' in 7.2 million or 4 per cent of the population (Hazell 1979b). These figures were based on a 'hearing status' survey undertaken between 1960 and 1962. These remain, according to Loavenbruck (1980), the only national data regarding the incidence of tinnitus in the general American population. A stratified sample of individuals was questioned about the presence and the severity of this condition. The incidence of tinnitus appeared to increase with age and appeared to occur more frequently in women than in men.

EARLY UK FIGURES

The prevalence of tinnitus was measured in 1957 and 1959 in random samples of adults drawn from rural populations in South Wales and in South-West Scotland as part of an investigation into the prevalence of the more common ear, nose and throat conditions (Hinchcliffe 1961). The prevalence of a history of tinnitus, based on self-reports given at otological and audiometric examinations, was 21 per cent in people as young as 18 to 24 years and went up to 39 per cent in people aged over 55. These figures would be lower if tinnitus of very short duration was excluded from them.

INSTITUTE OF HEARING RESEARCH ESTIMATES

These estimates were based on a brief postal questionnaire sent out as part of a pilot study to a random sample of some 7000 adults from the population in Cardiff, Glasgow, Nottingham and Southampton and this was followed by physical examination of a stratified sub-sample of those who responded. In this study head noises of less than five minutes duration were excluded, as were noises occurring just after loud sounds, e.g. discos, shooting or noise at work. From this study Coles *et al.* (1981) reported a prevalence (of tinnitus that was more than momentary or merely temporary after exposure to noise) of betwen 15.5 and 18.6 per cent in the populations of the four cities studied. It would appear from this study, then, that overall some 17 per cent of the UK population may have tinnitus, of whom 5 per cent might report severe annoyance from it, and 0.5 per cent may have tinnitus that has a very severe effect upon their life — on some to the extent that they could not carry on working or engage in social activities. Generalised to the population of the UK as a whole, these incidence figures suggest that there may be some 200,000 adults for whom tinnitus severely effects their ability to lead a normal life, and about four million for whom tinnitus causes moderate or severe annoyance and/or interference with getting to sleep (Coles 1983). In the USA perhaps as many as one million or more adults have tinnitus that has a very severe effect on their lives.

Other findings of interest from this study concerned age at onset, sex of respondent and the occupational classification of the respondent. As far as the latter is concerned, the prevalence of tinnitus in non-manual occupations was 8.7 per cent, which was half that for those in manual occupations (17.2 per cent) and much less than other occupational groups (comprising unemployed persons, housewives, and retired people) for whom the prevalence figure was 20 per cent. As far as age is concerned, the study showed it to be a major factor, there being markedly more tinnitus in the older age groups. To what extent this is due to ageing *per se* and due also to longer exposure to noise, remains to be explained, although Coles (1984b) suggests the effects are additive and independent.

Many of today's elderly had no opportunity to indulge in the acoustic indiscretions of today's youth, but many will have experienced adverse environmental noise in factory and other industrial work settings, as well as in two world wars. Interestingly, the Institute of Hearing Research study suggests that if anything women report tinnitus rather more often than do men. Coles (1981) expresses surprise at this finding since he considers men will tend to have had more noise exposure. Coles considers that one explanation may be that there are sex differences in attitudes to bodily disorders, suggesting that, perhaps, the prevalence among women is the same as for men, but women are more likely to be aware of it and/or report it.

The Institute of Hearing Research pilot study goes some way to indicate the prevalence of tinnitus that might obtain in the UK. But as Coles *et al.* (1981) points out, a much larger sample is required to estimate prevalence figures to the degree of precision required for detailed administrative action. Nevertheless they suggest that a quarter of a million people in the UK with tinnitus may need specialised help beyond that provided by their family doctor.

GENERAL HOUSEHOLD SURVEY FIGURES

The General Household Survey data for 1981 (Office of Population Censuses and Surveys, 1983) goes some considerable way to providing a statistically valid national estimate of the prevalence of tinnitus and is based on personal interviews undertaken with more than 23,000 individuals aged 16 or over.

Prevalence of tinnitus in the UK, 1981

The survey authors acknowledge that without taking a medical history (something usually undertaken by a medical professional), establishing the presence or absence of a subjective symptom by using a structured interview schedule (and trained — but not medically trained — interviewers) poses some difficulty.

Overall some 22 per cent of the adults interviewed said they had heard noises in their heads or ears such as ringing or buzzing sounds. It appeared that some noises were brought on by such things as colds or catarrh, water in the ears or by loud sounds, in one-third of these respondents. This third were removed from further analysis of the data as they were considered not to have tinnitus as conventionally defined.

Thus, 15 per cent of the sample reported hearing noises in the head or ears of a kind not due to known external stimuli, i.e. between 1 in 6 and 1 in 7 of the adult population of the UK. Two people in every 100 interviewed reported that they heard noises in their head or ears *continuously*. Roughly two-thirds of those with tinnitus said that there was nothing specific that brought it on — its appearance was quite unpredictable. Those who could name something that appeared to start the tinnitus off (some one-third of those with tinnitus), mentioned such things as stress, tiredness, particular medical conditions or simply lying in bed at night.

Severity of the tinnitus

Of the 15 per cent of the entire sample who reported tinnitus, just under one in seven said the noise was continuous and one in eight said it occurred daily or nearly every day even though it wasn't continuous. Five in ten of those with tinnitus heard the noises on average less than once a week. One in three respondents with tinnitus said the noise lasted less than a minute but less than half an hour. Some of these respondents would have been excluded from the Institute of Hearing Research incidence figures for people with tinnitus on the grounds that they typically experienced tinnitus for a duration of less than five minutes. When the frequency with which tinnitus occurred was taken, together with the length of time for which it usually appeared, as an indication of 'severity' (although the nature of the noise and its perceived loudness must obviously influence 'severity' too), about one in five of those with tinnitus heard noises every day or nearly every day, for all or most of the day. This represents 'severe' tinnitus in roughly three in every 100 members of the adult population of the UK at large.

Quality of life

About two in every 100 adults in the general population appeared to have noises that bothered them quite a lot or a great deal. Not surprisingly the more continuous the tinnitus was, the more likely respondents with tinnitus were to say that it bothered them. About one-third of those with tinnitus (five in every 100 of the general population) said that at one time or another they had consulted a doctor about it, and the more the noises bothered the individual the more he or she was likely to have consulted a doctor about them. Nearly one in five of those whose tinnitus bothered them a great deal had consulted a doctor about it within the month prior to the survey interview. Even among this group — those bothered a great deal — one in four had never seen a doctor about the tinnitus.

Age, sex and tinnitus prevalence

About one in eight people in the general population aged 16 to 44 years reported tinnitus, but this rose to one in five of the general population aged 65 and older. In each age group tinnitus was more common among women than men.

Occupation and tinnitus prevalence

The age composition of the population working in different occupational groups itself differs, and since age and tinnitus prevalence is associated it is necessary to remove this influence when attempting to examine the association between occupation and tinnitus incidence. This done, it appeared that one in ten of the general population working in professional occupations reports tinnitus whereas just more than one in five of those in manual work does. Again in each occupational level tinnitus appeared to be more common among women than among men.

Tinnitus and ill health

Removing the effects of the age of respondent on the incidence figures reveals that for all age groups tinnitus is associated with other measures of ill-health included in the General Household Survey. Those who reported long-standing illness, disability or infirmity were twice as likely to have tinnitus as those who reported no such long-standing sickness. In a similar vein, those respondents who reported that illness had restricted their activities in the two weeks prior to the survey interview were more likely to report tinnitus (22 per cent) than those not so restricted (14 per cent).

Incidence figures — a summary

The Institute of Hearing Research figures suggest that tinnitus has a severe deleterious effect on the quality of life of one in every 200 adults in the UK — perhaps these are the true 'sufferers'. In a letter to the *Guardian* newspaper (15 February 1983) Prof. Mark Haggard suggests that the General Household Survey figures, by presenting the number of people 'reporting tinnitus' as 15 per cent of the UK adult population, may mislead people into over-estimating the scope of the problem. Tinnitus is not a problem for the large majority of people who 'report it' when questioned. The General Household Survey suggests that three in every 100 individuals have a more-or-less continuous tinnitus, and that some two in every 100 individuals in the general population have tinnitus that bothers them a great deal or quite a lot. The figure of 0.5 per cent with 'significant disturbance' due to the tinnitus may be taken as being the more conservative and the less potentially alarmist. Nevertheless it reveals a large

Table 6.1: Likely number of 'true tinnitus sufferers'[a] in selected major cities

City	Number of likely 'sufferers'[b]
Greater London	33,800
Cardiff	1400
Edinburgh	2100
Manchester	2200
Liverpool	2500
New York	33,300
San Francisco	3300
Boston	2800
Minneapolis	1800
Ottawa	3500
Calgary	2900
Halifax, N.S.	1300
Paris	11,400
Strasbourg	1200
Hamburg	8100
Cologne	4800
Leipzig	2800

Note: a. a 'true tinnitus sufferer' is taken from Institute of Hearing Research UK prevalence figures as one person per 200 adult population.
b. The figures have been rounded down to the nearest hundred.
Source: Original population statistics are taken from the Europa Year Book (1984 and 1983), Europa Publications Ltd.

number of individuals with a reduced quality of life due to tinnitus.

Table 6.1 indicates how many 'true tinnitus sufferers' might exist in various major cities.

HEARING IMPAIRMENT AND THE INCIDENCE OF TINNITUS

The General Household Survey figures clearly suggest that tinnitus is associated with hearing impairment. Four in ten of the general population using a hearing aid reported tinnitus. Of those in the general population who had no aid but nevertheless reported hearing difficulties, tinnitus was reported by one person in three. This compares with tinnitus reported by one in ten of those who say they have no hearing difficulty. As the General Household Survey report suggests, this may partly explain the association between the prevalence of tinnitus and age and occupation, since hearing impairment is more common among older people and among those in manual occupations.

Others have commented on the association of tinnitus and

95

deafness. Coles *et al.* (1981) report finding that half of their sample with tinnitus had some hearing loss. As Douek points out in the same paper, many individuals with tinnitus may not be aware of the fact that they *do* have mild forms of high-tone hearing loss, i.e. self reports on matters of this nature need confirming by more objective evidence where possible and available. Even then, conventionally used audiometers for assessing hearing acuity may themselves not be capable of revealing a sufficiently fine-grained profile of hearing loss and McFadden (1982) suggests that it may be preferable to assume that *all* tinnitus sufferers have *some* hearing loss. This remains a somewhat contentious assertion. It is likely that figures showing the prevalence of hearing impairment among people with tinnitus will be under-estimated rather than over-estimated. Another way of presenting the information is to consider that two out of every three individuals with moderate or severe hearing loss may have tinnitus. Obviously for many individuals hearing loss with tinnitus represents a double stress.

Three musicians

We noted earlier that an attempt would be made to put a 'human face' to the figures, where possible. Here we consider the influence tinnitus had on Beethoven, Schumann and Smetana.

Beethoven (1770–1827)

The following extract is taken from Edward Larkin's medical appendix to Martin Cooper's 'Beethoven — the Last Decade' (1970, p. 440).

Beethoven's deafness is clearly of such importance that it should be described first. It started somewhere about his twenty-eighth year when he had already written the first symphony, the first two piano concertos, and the sonatas up to op. 13, and had done most of the work on the string quartets of op. 18. He first admitted to it in his thirty-first year, i.e. about the end of his 'first period'. It was progressive but with periods of standstill. It was accompanied by incessant noises, ringing, whistling and rushing. There were ear-aches and head-aches for the rest of his life, the ear-aches being particularly troublesome every February, the depth of winter. The upper tones were lost first and loud jarring noises were very painful. 'Sometimes I can scarcely hear a person who speaks softly; I can hear sound, it is true, but cannot make out the words. But if anyone shouts, I can't bear it.' (1801) During the bombardment of Vienna (1809) he went to the cellar and covered his ears with cushions: even in his fifties he sometimes had to have cotton wool in his ears in noisy surroundings.

Schumann (1810–1856)

The following extract is taken from Marcel Brion's 'Schumann and the Romantic Age' (1956, pp. 345, 350 and 351).

'The music is hushed, at all events outwardly . . .' ‐

With these words to Joachim [a musician and violinist], Schumann took his leave of the music written on staves. Henceforth he would listen to that 'other music', that terrible language which the devils and the angels would from now on pour into his ear.

For some time now, Schumann and those around him had been alarmed by certain symptoms — auditive disorders and difficulty of speech. Becher, the violinist, relates how one evening in a cafe Schumann put down the newspaper he had been reading saying: 'I can't read any more. I keep hearing the note A'. The troubles were temporary, generally lasting a few days, after which Schumann would be brighter and gayer than usual, because greatly relieved; for he was obsessed with the fear they might become chronic. Seeing Brahms or Joachim always cheered him up and enabled him to go on composing or working at a Dichtergarten, but during the night of 10th–11th February, 1854, he suffered so intolerably as to be quite unable to sleep. A few days before, he had ended his last letter to Joachim with those terrible words: 'It is already beginning to be night'. It was this letter which contained that enigmatic remark whose meaning was probably known only to himself; '. . . and between the lines there is yet another secret message which will be revealed later'. This feeling that darkness was crowding round him, and that terrible note that rang in his ears for hours on end provoked a mortal anguish of mind all the more unbearable for being accompanied by perfect lucidity.

Smetana (1824–1884)

The following extract is taken from Frantisek Bartos' book

'Bedvrich Smetana — Letters and Reminiscences' (1953, pp. 147, 189, 190, 212).

Smetana's Diary, July, 1874

28th. My hearing is failing and at the same time my head seems to be spinning and I feel giddy. It started during a short duck-shooting expedition. The weather had changed suddenly just before.

. . . As regards the style of my first string quartet, I gladly leave others to judge, and I shall not be in the least angry if this style does not find favour or is considered contrary to what was hitherto regarded as quartet style. I did not intend to write a quartet according to recipe and according to custom in the usual forms. As a young apprentice in music theory I worked sufficiently hard to acquire thorough knowledge and mastery of them. With me the form of every composition is given by the subject itself. And thus this quartet, took, shaped its form itself. I had wanted to give a tone picture of my life. First movement: My leaning towards art in my youth, the romantic atmosphere, the inexpressible longing for something I could neither express nor define and also the presage, as it were, of my future misfortune and the long, insistent note, the one in the Finale, etc. grew out of this beginning. It is that fateful ringing of high-pitched tones in my ear which in 1874 announced the beginning of my deafness. I allowed myself this little play because for me it was so prophetic.

To the question whether it did not tire him to look through the new scores of others, he would answer: 'No; when I look at the written music it comes to life in my imagination without any effort of will on my part, as though I could really hear the instruments and voices; only if I persist for some time, then I feel a most unpleasant vibration in my head and the ringing increases . . . That ringing in my head That noise!' the unhappy master would complain '. . . that is worst of all. Deafness would be a relatively decent condition if only all was quiet in my head. But the greatest torture is caused me by the almost continuous internal noise which goes on in my head and sometimes rises to a thunderous crashing'.

7

When Tinnitus Starts

CHILDHOOD ONSET — THE PRESENT STUDY

The notion that children more readily accept symptoms may partly explain the interesting phenomenon brought to the first author's attention by members of his local tinnitus self-help group. At the first meeting one woman aged 26 reported that she had had tinnitus for as long as she could remember, but that for years she had simply assumed that everyone else had it too — that it was perfectly normal. It was not until she was in her teens that it gradually dawned on her that other people didn't have it. At the same meeting a middle-aged man reported that he had only discovered his 14-year-old daughter had had tinnitus for as long as she could remember, when he himself started to suffer with it and complained about it.

In our survey of 984 individuals with tinnitus, two respondents reported being as young as three when they *first* noticed that they had tinnitus in any form that lasted for a long time, and 2.6 per cent of the sample said the onset of their tinnitus occurred when they were under ten years old. All in all some 10 per cent considered that the tinnitus had started before they reached their 21st birthday.

A study by Nodar (1972), in which 6000 school children (aged ten to 18) in New York were investigated with routine audiometric screening procedures over a three-year period, revealed an overall incidence of tinnitus of 15 per cent which rose to 58 per cent in the group that failed an auditory screening test. The most common characterisations of the tinnitus, by those who passed *and* by those who failed the audiometric screening, were 'high' and 'ringing', which suggests either a common type of tinnitus or a common type of mechanism causing the tinnitus (Nodar and LeZak 1984). In another study of hearing-impaired children, Nodar and LeZak (1984) reported that 49 of 56 children examined had tinnitus that could be matched to a pure tone rather than to a band of frequencies.

AGE OF ONSET

Although tinnitus obviously *can* start in childhood, or even infancy, the most common period of life for its onset appears to be in middle age — around the time of the real menopause in women and the so-called menopause (mid-life crisis?) in men. Shulman (1981a) refers to its 'menopausal peak in the male', and directs attention to the importance and distinguishing characteristics of middle age. Hazell (1979c) reporting his intensive study of 200 tinnitus sufferers, notes a curious finding, namely that subjects with tinnitus in their left ear showed a much higher incidence of onset of the condition in middle-age than those with tinnitus in the right ear, whose age of onset was more evenly distributed through the age groups. Overall, though, the commonest age of onset for his subjects was in the 50 to 60 year-old range, which, if anything, is a rather late menopausal peak. It has been suggested that one underlying factor (of several) may be that some people do become depressed and introspective around the menopause, and this may cause them to take note of a symptom that might have gone largely unnoticed for some time.

Age of onset in the present study

Whereas the youngest age of onset reported in our study, by two respondents, was age three, the oldest age of onset was 88! Table 7.1 gives age of onset in ten-year age bands.

Although the average age of onset was just under 45 years of age, the occurrence of tinnitus would appear to rise sharply in the 40- to 49-year-old group, peaking in the 50- to 59-year-old group. If you are going to get tinnitus it would seem there is a 50/50 chance it will start between age 40 and 59.

Table 7.1 Age of onset of tinnitus in ten-year age bands

Age group	Per cent
Age under 19	8.2
20 to 29	10.6
30 to 39	13.8
40 to 49	21.1
50 to 59	28.5
60 to 69	14.2
Aged 70 or over	3.5

Source: The present study — based on 960 respondents.

Possible reasons for age of onset

There are several possible factors that might be jointly at work in helping to produce a peak in tinnitus onset in middle age. One is a *delayed* response to damage done in earlier years; another is accumulated noise exposure; there is also ageing *per se* to be considered along with the associated disorder of the hearing mechanism — presbyacusis. Accumulated exposure to certain drugs may potentially be implicated in some cases.

Drug exposure

With age (and ultimately growing infirmity) there is an increasing likelihood that drugs which are known to be able to damage the hearing mechanism, whether that of particularly sensitive individuals or people in general, will have been consumed, or may have been consumed periodically over extended periods of time. The aches and pains that might start in middle age, such as back aches, may be relieved by aspirin consumption, which could induce tinnitus in certain susceptible individuals. Furthermore, it is theoretically possible that drug exposure and noise exposure may have potentiating effects the one upon the other — that is, both together may do more damage than the total damage if both occurred separately (Brown, Penny, Henley, Hodges, Kupetz, Glenn and Jobe 1981).

Noise exposure

We noted earlier the remark by Coles *et al.* (1981) about tinnitus of middle age onset possibly being initiated by 'acoustic indiscretions of youth' as well as by industrial noise exposure and accumulated exposure to the domestic and recreational hazards of modern life. They also note that those with transient tinnitus *now* may be those who get more constant tinnitus 20 years hence. Hazell (1979b) notes that there is in certain instances a clear causal relation between acoustic trauma and tinnitus, although the onset of tinnitus may be years after the exposure.

Ageing and associated hearing disorders

With ageing there come various alterations in the structure of the inner ear. Suffice it to say here that an important membrane (the basilar membrane), which vibrates in response to external sound, thickens and becomes less pliant, and cells thought to play a major role in the process of changing sound signals into electrical nerve impulses (the hair cells) degenerate. There may be degeneration in

101

the blood supply and disruptive pockets of fluid may form in other important cell sytems (e.g. in the spiral ganglion cells; Turner 1982). *Presbyacusis* is the medical term given to the changes that impair hearing and are solely due to the ageing process. Turner points out, though, that older patients are often *misdiagnosed* as having presbyacusis, as opposed to other hearing disorders, and comprehensive audiometry should be carried out to see if the hearing loss is due to *conductive* incapacity of the bones in the middle ear rather than to changes due to ageing in the inner ear. It is likely that some of the damage involved in presbyacusis can be a causative agent in the production of tinnitus in some people. One of the annoying aspects of presbyacusis that may be exacerbated by the presence of tinnitus is that the ability to hear high-pitched sounds is most affected, so that consonants (e.g. p, b, or r) are not distinguished though vowel sounds can still be heard. This often means that speech seems to be unclear and difficult to understand.

Otosclerosis is another disorder of the ear, and though it is an hereditary defect often developing in late adolescence and is not due to the ageing process itself, it nevertheless tends to be more common later rather than earlier in life. In this disorder the bones in the middle ear that transmit sounds from the ear drum and the outside world to the inner ear (the cochlea) become less mobile because of the formation of superfluous bone. Though harmless in most cases, if the abnormal bone blocks transmission to the inner ear, hearing is lost. The low-frequency 'rushing' tinnitus associated with otosclerosis may sometimes be helped by surgery. Otosclerosis does not necessarily always have tinnitus as a concomitant — the two disorders are common enough for both conditions to exist 'independently' i.e. with separate causes, in many individuals, although House (1981a) notes that tinnitus *is* a common complaint of patients with otosclerosis. Thomas and Cody (1981) point out that otosclerosis is generally easy to diagnose in patients with a normal ear drum (precluding middle ear disease), and it is suggested by a triad of symptoms — deafness, tinnitus and balance problems. Shea (1981) points out that its treatment is problematic as far as tinnitus is concerned. The otosclerotic process can affect the inner as well as the middle ear and Shea warns surgeons not to imply to the patient that the tinnitus will be relieved by surgery. The stapedectomy operation for otosclerosis (in which the third middle ear bone is replaced by a tiny plastic piston) is very unpredictable as far as its effect on tinnitus is concerned (Robinson 1984).

Age of onset — some results from the present study

If factors contributing to the emergence of tinnitus as a symptom are in any way additive, one might hypothesise that respondents who have experienced noise exposure might have an earlier onset of tinnitus than those who have had no similar experience. We asked our respondents 'Have you ever worked in an extremely noisy place where conversation was impossible even when shouting?' An analysis of the average age of onset for those who replied 'yes' and those who replied 'no' showed no statistically significant difference — the mean age of onset in both groups being about 45. A similar question asking 'Have you ever worked in a noisy office or factory where conversation was difficult and had to be conducted by shouting?' produced identical results — no difference in mean age between the two groups. When respondents who had worked for six or more years where it was impossible to converse even when shouting were compared with those who had experienced five years or less of such exposure, no differences in age of onset of tinnitus were found. A similar analysis comparing those who had worked nine or more years in conditions where it was difficult to converse with those who had experienced less of such exposure again revealed no difference in age of onset of tinnitus.

The absence of any significant difference in age of onset associated with noise exposure at work may explain why no difference was found between age of onset in males and females, although the incidence figures referred to earlier suggest that tinnitus may be slightly more common in women and hence that women may be more susceptible. Men in our sample were more likely than one would have expected on a chance basis than the women to have worked in conditions where it was impossible or difficult to converse, supporting Coles' (1981) contention that males will tend to have had more noise exposure than women.

If women *are* more susceptible than men, but men have had more noise exposure, the two effects may cancel giving similar age of onset figures for each sex. However, no sex differences in mean age of onset of tinnitus were found among respondents who had answered 'no' to the two questions about working in noisy conditions, and similarly no sex differences were found in mean age of onset of tinnitus among respondents who answered 'yes', indicating that they *had* had some experience of working in a noisy environment. From our study, then, there is no evidence that sex is a factor influencing age of onset — although this is, of course, not to say it plays no part in influencing the prevalence figures. In any event the lack of any differences in age of onset according to previous noise exposure remains intriguing. It is possible that different causative factors are at work in the two groups, each of which tends to lead to tinnitus peaking in middle age.

Although noise exposure did not appear to be linked to age of onset, occupational level did, and in a surprising way. Those in manual occupations clearly had had significantly more experience of working in noisy environments than had non-manual respondents, yet the mean age of onset of tinnitus among respondents whose occupation was classified into one of three manual categories was 48.6 compared with 43.3 for respondents from non-manual occupations. (This difference is statistically quite significant — $P < 0.001$.) The result is counter-intuitive — one might have expected, if anything, that manual workers (with more experience of noise exposure) would have had tinnitus earlier than non-manual workers. Given the lack of difference in age of onset according to noise exposure, one must ask what is it about respondents in manual occupations that may facilitate a later age of onset of tinnitus? Table 7.2 gives a more detailed breakdown of age of onset of tinnitus among respondents in manual and non-manual occupations.

If age of onset is at least *partially* indicative of susceptibility to tinnitus, it would appear that those in non-manual occupations may be more susceptible than respondents in manual occupations. It is possible, however, that those who work in relatively quiet surroundings are more likely to actually *notice* that they have tinnitus, particularly if it is, at onset, of a quiet or otherwise unobtrusive form, and this seems the most likely explanation of the above results.

Respondents were asked if they had ever been close to an explosion, extremely loud noises or gunfire, and if so did it happen regularly at some time in their life. No mean age of onset differences were found between those with no experience of explosions, etc., and those with such experience, nor did the regularity of this happening relate to differences in mean age of tinnitus onset. Respondents were also asked in our survey if they had ever gone regularly to discos and/or loud rock concerts at some time in their life. When the sample was restricted to those aged 50 or under, i.e. the generations most likely to have had the opportunity of attending such events since their youth, a significant difference in age of onset of tinnitus was found. Age at tinnitus onset was 33.2 years for those 176 individuals who had never gone regularly to discos and/or loud rock concerts, but was 37.9 for those 35 persons who had ($t = 3.05$,

Table 7.2: Age of onset of tinnitus by manual and non-manual occupations

Age group	% Non-Manual	% Manual
Age under 19	9.8	2.2
20 to 29	12.0	8.1
30 to 39	15.1	14.8
40 to 49	20.4	19.3
50 to 59	27.4	33.3
60 to 69	12.3	18.5
Aged 70 or over	3.0	3.7
Total	100	100
Number of Respondents	569	135
		$(\chi^2 = 13.6,\ df = 6,\ P = 0.033)$

Source: The present study.

$df = 55,\ P = 0.003$). This is a somewhat surprising and counter-intuitive difference in age of onset of tinnitus, especially considering the lack of any similar differences in age of onset between other groups with different levels of exposure to other forms of environmental noise.

We mentioned earlier a curious result reported by Hazell (1979c), that among those with tinnitus whom he studied, those with tinnitus in the left ear showed a very much higher incidence of the onset of the condition between ages 50 and 60, whereas the age of onset for those with tinnitus in the right ear was more evenly distributed throughout the age groups. In connection with this finding he noted that tinnitus may be related to cerebral blood flow and to hemispherical dominance, i.e. which side of the two halves of the brain seems most dominant under certain conditions. Of his sample he also noted that all patients who were diagnosed as having tinnitus due to interference with the blood supply in one way or another (vascular insufficiency) had tinnitus in their left ear. Hazell seems to be suggesting that vascular insufficiency may be more likely to produce tinnitus in the left ear, and that this condition may itself have a prevalence peak among people aged 50 to 59. We were unable to reproduce Hazell's findings exactly from the data in our study. Simply comparing those respondents who had stated the tinnitus was in their left ear with those who said it was in their right ear (at the present time) revealed no significant difference in the mean age of onset. Table 7.3 gives a more detailed breakdown of age of onset by present tinnitus location.

Despite there being no difference in the *mean* age of onset of

Table 7.3: Age of onset of tinnitus by current location of tinnitus

| Age group | Location of tinnitus | | | |
	Left ear %	Right ear %	Both ears %	Within the head %
Age under 19	6.5	3.6	11.5	8.6
20 to 29	11.2	7.9	13.9	8.8
30 to 39	11.2	16.4	13.2	15.0
40 to 49	23.7	27.1	19.8	17.3
50 to 59	32.1	22.1	26.4	31.0
60 to 69	11.2	17.1	13.5	15.7
Aged 70 and over	4.2	5.7	1.7	3.6
Total	100	100	100	100
Number of respondents	215	140	288	306

$(\chi^2 = 32.37, df = 18, P = 0.02)$

Source: The present study.

tinnitus according to its present location, it would appear that location and age of onset are not completely independent of one another. In our sample, tinnitus onset peaked in the age 50 to 59 range for those with tinnitus presently in the left, in both ears, or within the head, whereas onset peaked in the 40 to 49 age range for those with tinnitus in the right ear. Several analyses examining whether mean age of tinnitus onset differed according to current tinnitus location failed to show significant differences — except one. This revealed that those respondents whose tinnitus was currently in both their ears or in their head had an earlier mean onset age for tinnitus, 43.9, than those whose tinnitus was apparently in the left or the right ear only, who had a mean onset age of 46.1. It may be the case that those who get tinnitus in both ears tend to have more susceptibility to it and hence may get it earlier.

It could also be the case that tinnitus in both ears or within the head is perceived as louder, other things being equal, than tinnitus at only one ear. This makes intuitive sense since noises in both ears might be expected to feel louder than noise in only one. Analysis of our survey data showed that, when rating their present tinnitus on a nine-point scale of loudness (quiet = 1, 9 = extremely loud), those with tinnitus in both ears or within the head *did* rate the tinnitus as louder (mean scale score 3.9), but only marginally so, than those whose present tinnitus was considered by respondents to be in one ear only (mean scale score 3.5, $t = -3.07, df = 798, P = 0.002$). If anything tinnitus located *within* the head appeared to be louder than that in one or in both ears, when the nine-point scale was used as an indicator of loudness.

INITIAL REACTIONS AND MEDIATING FACTORS

As yet there are no readily available generalisable survey data documenting how individuals tend to react to the onset of tinnitus. But there are several factors in the situation that arguably will influence their reactions. These are: the nature of the tinnitus; the suddenness or otherwise of its appearance; the age of the individual; and concurrent stress factors.

The nature of the tinnitus

Some tinnitus sounds are, obviously, intrinsically worse than others, be it in their apparent loudness, pitch, variety, timbre, etc. The sound that chalk can make when it 'squeaks' against a blackboard, would, for example, be more unendurable than a low 'hiss' or 'rumble'. Consider the following description of an individual with tinnitus, sent in a letter from one specialist to another:

> Thank you very much for asking me to see this patient whom I have no doubt has about the worst tinnitus I have seen. This dates back to a bomb injury in 1946, and his hearing and tinnitus became increasingly worse as time went on. The worst tinnitus is in the left ear and takes the form of multiple sounds which are hissing, screaming, squealing and pulsating and are at their very lowest at the same level of intensity as his own voice. Despite this he manages to sleep quite well, but they have affected his concentration quite severely and he is unable at the moment to carry on with his work. The most severe problem, for which he initially came to see you, was the sudden onset of a very loud sound in his head like a referee's whistle. This has continued non-stop since then and at one point he thought he was going quite mad.

Suddenness of onset

In about 40 per cent of cases the onset of tinnitus comes quite suddenly for no apparent reason. To the extent that onset *is* sudden —

'out of the blue' — the reaction to the tinnitus is likely to be the more distraught, particularly if the noise seems to be loud and/or unpleasant. As noted earlier: 'Many patients are convinced that the sudden onset or horrendous noise inside the head heralds haemorrhage, neoplasia [a tumour] or insanity, and who can blame them?' (Hazell 1979b)

Hallam, Rachman and Hinchcliffe (1984) suggest that sudden onset of tinnitus is more likely to precipitate complaint, assuming that gradual onset, to some extent at least, facilitates habituation — the ability not to notice sounds that are present, often at a constant continuous level, in the environment. Many people habituate to, i.e. get used to and don't notice any more, sounds such as distant motorway traffic noise or even the television on in the same room. Hallam *et al.* consider that, theoretically at least, individuals might be able to habituate to tinnitus.

Age of individual at onset

Onset of tinnitus in childhood may be more readily accepted, taken for granted even, under some circumstances, than it is in adulthood. Other things being equal it is likely that onset in young adulthood, in someone who otherwise considers him or herself to be 'young, healthy and fit' is harder for the individual to accept and cope with than it is for the person in retirement, say, who might already be aware of some hearing loss. Certainly the first author remembers well one young adult, recently started with tinnitus who desperately tried to find others her own age 'because only they will be able to understand what it's like to have it at my age'. While this was perhaps an uncharitable view of the misery that tinnitus can cause irrespective of the age of onset, the thought of 'carrying the burden' for 50 years might be more initially devastating than the thought of carrying it for ten.

Concurrent stress factors

There are probably more stress factors impinging on the elderly person than the young or middle aged. In later life, with declining health and physical and financial resources, more to worry about and less to gain satisfaction from, the onset of tinnitus might, in the event, be just as upsetting and debilitating as it is in a young adult.

We shall see later how stress plays a major role in facilitating the debilitating and annoying nature of tinnitus. Those already under pressure may well react to tinnitus as something of a 'last straw' and be less able to see it in proportion.

Feverish imaginations

Given, say, a piercing and loud tinnitus of sudden onset, the imagination of the sufferer does not have to be too feverish for a connection to be made between something producing a noise in his or her ears or head and something being 'wrong' in their head. Of course something *is* 'wrong', but most 'sufferers' will not be aware of the microscopic and otherwise insignificant changes that may take place at cell level to produce tinnitus, but rather will think of common causes for things going wrong in people's heads. As Hazell suggests, strokes, burst blood vessels, brain cancer, brain disease and deterioration, may cross the sufferer's mind as potential causes. Indeed, in extremely rare cases such may *be* the causes, but far too rare to worry about.

Despite the prevalence of tinnitus in the general population, the average family doctor may see for the first time as few as three individuals a year for whom tinnitus is their dominant complaint. This may be one reason why family doctors need reminding that what many patients need at first is strong re-assurance. House (see Goodey 1981), of the Otologic Medical Group in Los Angeles, states that 95 per cent of the patients who go to see him simply need an explanation of the problem as their solution to it — 'Once they know the source of the noise and why it is there, these patients are satisfied.' Hazell and Wood (1981) suggest that some one-third of patients attending a tinnitus clinic mainly require reassurance about their symptoms (following proper otological and audiological investigation); 5 per cent of all patients referred are amenable to various forms of medical or surgical treatment, and the remainder — some 62 per cent — are referred for a trial of masking. But does the person with sudden, or for that matter gradual, tinnitus onset get from family doctors and specialists the explanations and reassurances he or she deserves?

8

Onset Factors and Development

In this section we will examine the circumstances and events that 'trigger off' tinnitus and we will present our own respondents' ideas as to what they thought the onset of their tinnitus was connected with. It does not follow, of course, that what respondents *thought* the onset of tinnitus might be caused by or associated with in any way reflects the *actual* cause of the onset, were one actually able to ascertain it (which would be impossible in the majority of cases anyway).

TRIGGERS

In reply to a reader's letter the medical adviser to the BTA points out that the tinnitus that is triggered by certain sounds, though fairly common in his practice, is nevertheless a particular kind of tinnitus and that the reader's experience would not apply to the majority of tinnitus sufferers. The reader wrote:

> My very high pitched whistle varies from moderate to intolerable within a quarter of an hour and now takes a day, or more, to fade again. Noises of many kinds bring on my severe attacks, my best defence being to seek quiet environments and to use ear-plugs. Two particular items of modern living trigger a sharp increase in tinnitus level in both ears. The first is the proximity of a 625-line television set with or without the sound . . . The other trigger is almost all cars (BTA, 1984, p. 10).

In this case it appeared that the reader might be especially sensitive to low frequency sounds that he could not hear but that somehow triggered off an increase in the loudness of tinnitus. Walford (1980) also reports (rare) forms of tinnitus that he calls 'type 2 hums', in which the tinnitus is triggered by certain kinds of noises that are quite different from the tinnitus apparently being triggered. He gives examples of the chirping of birds triggering in some individuals tinnitus that sounds like a 'rustling click'. Triggers are not restricted to varieties of environmental noise. Again in a reply to a BTA reader's letter the medical adviser points out that many people with tinnitus have a history of extreme worry or anxiety or bereavement prior to the onset of the complaint, which may be a triggering factor in some cases.

SYRINGING AND WAX

Several readers of the BTA Newsletter have written asking if syringing wax from the ears can set off tinnitus. The medical adviser's reply has been that although patients have reported in the past that tinnitus occurred after ear syringing it is thought that this would be an initiating factor in the onset of tinnitus only in susceptible ears, i.e. in ears that are highly likely to produce tinnitus sooner or later. He points out that syringing has been responsible for the safe removal of wax and the restoration of hearing in thousands of cases but elsewhere notes that syringing an ear with a perforation often results in discharge and this is one reason why it is best not to syringe an ear with wax in it unless it has previously been established that the ear drum is intact.

Elsewhere the medical adviser points out that tinnitus can be caused by impacted wax that can be treated by a family doctor or at the local ENT clinic. He suggests that impacted wax is largely caused by the unfortunately widespread practice of individuals pushing cotton buds, corners of towels, fingers, and other objects down the ear in the mistaken belief that this is what is necessary to keep it clean. He suggests that 95 per cent of wax removal would be unnecessary if people refrained from doing this, and that only in 5 per cent of cases does wax need to be regularly removed by syringing because the ear's own cleaning mechanism is disordered. Just how wax might produce tinnitus was a point of discussion at the 85th Ciba Foundation Symposium:

Dr. Feldmann: Ear wax is often mentioned as a cause for tinnitus. In my experience it is only when the wax is attached to

111

the membrane [the drum] that it causes tinnitus and not if it just occludes [blocks off] the ear canal. It is probably a mechanical effect.

Dr. Coles: I would suggest that in those cases the tinnitus is 'revealed', and that there is an underlying sensorineural tinnitus [one due to changes in inner ear cell performance or in nerve conductivity]. This would cause sufficient conductive hearing loss [by making the middle ear bones less mobile] for the tinnitus sounds themselves to become audible, perhaps by reflection. When one removes the wax and the patient hears ambient noise normally again, he or she is no longer aware of the tinnitus. (Evered and Lawrenson, 1981, pp. 234–235)

We noted earlier that under some circumstances stress may trigger onset of tinnitus and we shall see in a later chapter how tinnitus seems to be influenced by stress. It may be worth pointing out here that factors that themselves influence stress and strain — viral infections, for example — may appear to trigger onset of tinnitus or changes in its loudness.

The questionnaire answered by the 984 respondents in our survey ended by asking: 'Is there anything else about your tinnitus which you would like to mention that was not asked in this questionnaire? If so, please tell us on the lines below.' And 14 blank lines were given for respondents to write on. Several filled the 14 lines and continued on extra sheets they supplied themselves. In many instances respondents answered by saying such things as 'I think my tinnitus may have been caused by . . .' or 'I think my tinnitus may be connected with . . .' These answers were coded and Table 8.1 summarises the analysis for the 114 relevant respondents.

Of those answering who speculated on what might have caused their tinnitus or with what its onset might have been connected, stress and loud noise are the predominant answers. Whether this would have been the case had respondents been asked direct questions about the likely cause for the tinnitus remains a matter of speculation.

The respondents' answers to the open question at the end of the questionnaire were also coded, where possible, into groups of answers dealing with events or circumstances that were concurrent with, or followed immediately after, the onset of the tinnitus, or which the respondent clearly thought actually caused the tinnitus. Table 8.2 summarises these responses.

Table 8.2 has been presented in detail to illustrate the variety of

Table 8.1: Tinnitus connected with/may have been caused by . . .

Speculative cause	Number	%	% Overall sample
Using ear-plugs	1	0.9	0.1
Wax in ear	7	6.1	0.7
Loud noise	27	23.5	2.7
Stress	26	22.6	2.6
Ear trouble	17	14.8	1.7
Catarrh/asthma	23	20.0	2.3
Migraine	3	2.6	0.3
Operation (not on ear)	7	6.1	0.7
Blow to ear or head	3	2.6	0.3
Total	114	100	(base = 984)

Source: The present study.

Table 8.2: Events concurrent with, immediately following, or 'causing' onset of tinnitus

Concurrent/'causative' factors	Number	%	% Overall sample
Loud noise	24	9.5	2.4
Menière's/vertigo	24	9.5	2.4
Bad cold, flu	32	12.6	3.3
Ear got very cold	1	0.4	0.1
High dive badly executed	1	0.4	0.1
Drugs, injections	22	8.7	2.2
'Blocked ears' (catarrh, wax)	13	5.1	1.3
Began without warning	28	11.1	2.8
Ear operation, infection	22	8.7	2.2
Blow to head or ear	20	7.9	2.0
Burst ear drum	7	2.8	0.7
Illness	18	7.1	1.8
Shock, stress	9	3.6	0.9
LSD trip	1	0.4	0.1
Menopause	2	0.8	0.2
Pregnancy	2	0.8	0.2
With deafness	22	8.7	2.2
Ear syringed/tooth drilled or taken out	5	2.0	0.5
Total	253	100	(base = 984)

Source: The present study.

events or circumstances that are clearly associated in respondents' minds with the onset of their tinnitus. It will never be clear which of these factors *did* play a causative role in the appearance of the individual's tinnitus. Many, if not most, may well be purely coincidental.

113

Most of the overall sample did not respond to the question in ways that could be coded as information about onset factors. For many of them onset may not have been attributable to anything specific. Overall, though, about one in eight respondents did produce answers suggesting they thought onset of tinnitus was connected with something specifiable; and one in four respondents clearly thought certain events or circumstances played a more causal role in initiating the tinnitus.

Since individual susceptibilities will be many and varied, in some cases a particular event (the LSD trip, say) may have initiated the tinnitus in a particular individual; but it far from follows that the same experience would produce tinnitus in others.

An attempt was made to see if the speculative causes for onset of tinnitus were associated with the sex or age of the respondent, his or her experience with noise, or his or her occupational level. The latter three factors revealed no interesting associations. There did appear to be some slight sex differences, however. Perhaps not unexpectedly, men were more likely than women to attribute onset to exposure to loud noise. Women seemed more likely than men to attribute onset to stress and to a bad cold or flu.

PROGRESSION FROM ONSET

Perhaps the most dominant question in the mind of the person who has recently begun to have tinnitus, and in particular for those whose onset was sudden and whose noise is continuous and inherently unpleasant, is, is it going to carry on like this or get worse, or is there a chance it will go? In the next section we will present what others have suggested is the likely outcome over time (prognosis) as well as the likelihood of the tinnitus going as suddenly as it may have come (spontaneous remission). We shall also present our own survey data as to how respondents reported their tinnitus had evolved since its onset.

PROGNOSIS AND REMISSION

There are no reliable figures that are nationally valid and available to enable a firm answer to be given to the general question concerning how tinnitus, once evident, will evolve. The medical adviser to the British Tinnitus Association suggests that the chances of recovery spontaneously from tinnitus are quite small, once it has become established for a period of, say, six months, and also if the tinnitus is more or less continuous. If the tinnitus is like that reported by many of the respondents in the General Household Survey (GHS), that is it is of an *intermittent* type (about half of those in the GHS with tinnitus heard noises less than once a week), and if it is of *short duration* (about one-third of those in the GHS with tinnitus said it lasted less than a minute when it occurred, and nearly another third said it lasted a few minutes but less than half an hour), there is a slightly increased chance of spontaneous recovery — put at less than one in ten. The chance of spontaneous recovery for the 15 per cent of those in the GHS with tinnitus whose tinnitus was of a continuous nature appears much lower. For all forms of tinnitus, the likelihood of spontaneous remission may be about one in 20, with nine of ten cases staying very much the same. However, when considering those with intermittent tinnitus of short duration, we must remember that some people with spontaneous momentary tinnitus *now* may be those who develop more continuous tinnitus in 20 years time (Coles *et al.* 1981). At the moment our general level of knowledge about tinnitus prognosis is far from complete, especially for those whose tinnitus is intermittent and/or of short duration. According to the General Household Survey data, 2 per cent of the population of Great Britain (aged 16 and over) have forms of tinnitus that are *continuous*, whereas 10 per cent have discontinuous forms that can be brought on at any time with no obvious cause and 3 per cent have discontinuous forms that they feel *are* brought on by something specific (OPCS, 1983).

PROGNOSIS FOR LOUDNESS — THE PRESENT STUDY

One element in the degree to which tinnitus gives annoyance, and effecting the ability of the individual to cope with it, is the perceived loudness of the tinnitus. 'Sufferers' often ask 'Will it get any louder the longer I have it?' or 'Does it get worse the older you are?' In our survey we asked respondents with tinnitus to make two ratings of loudness, the first being on an 'adjectival' scale as follows: 'Please put a tick alongside *one* phrase in the list below which best suggests the normal loudness of the tinnitus.' This list of phrases then followed: sound of your own breathing, whisper, water simmering on a pot, normal conversation, traffic noise in a busy street, thunderclap overhead, and low-flying jet aircraft. The second rating of loudness was ascertained thus: 'Please also indicate the loudness of the tinnitus on the following scale by circling *one* of the numbers below.'

1	2	3	4	5	6	7	8	9
Quiet		Moderately loud		Loud		Very loud		Extremely loud

An attempt was then made to see if the ratings given on these scales were associated with the length of time the respondents had had tinnitus, and the age of the respondent. Since we wished to look at these two factors independently (because the older you are the more time you've had in which to have had tinnitus longer) we undertook a statistical routine (a partial correlation) that would give us an indication of whether or not tinnitus tended to get rated as louder the longer people had it — independently of their age — and whether it tended to be rated louder the older the respondent was — independently of the length of time they had had the tinnitus. The results from over 900 respondents suggested that there was an association between tinnitus loudness and the length of time the respondent had tinnitus, it tending to get louder over time, as measured on the adjectival scale irrespective of the age of the respondents, and that this association, though weak, was unlikely to be due to chance factors ($n = 907$, $r = 0.103$, $P = 0.001$). This indicates that for by no means everyone will the tinnitus tend to be rated louder the longer that they have it, but that the trend is in that direction. However, the difference in rated loudness over time is slight enough not to be of worry for the vast majority of those with tinnitus. The mean rating of loudness on the adjectival scale for those who had had tinnitus for ten years or less was 3.6 (i.e. just over mid-way between the 'moderately loud' rating of 3 and the rating of 4), whereas the rating for those who had had tinnitus for more than ten years was just fractionally below the rating of 4.

An analysis showing the effect of age on loudness irrespective of the length of time the respondent had had tinnitus showed similar results. The tendency for tinnitus to be rated louder with increasing age was evident. Though the association was slight, it was not likely to be due to chance ($n = 907$, $r = 0.084$, $P = 0.006$). Again this finding need not worry the individual with tinnitus. The mean adjectival scale rating for respondents aged 60 or younger was 3.6, rising only to 3.9 for those 61 years or older; hardly a dramatic increase in perceived loudness! The range of loudness rating rose from a mean of 3.4 in those aged 39 or younger to 3.9 in those aged

60 to 70 years. For those aged 70 years or older the mean scale rating for loudness dropped to 3.8.

The weak association between age and the length of time a person has had tinnitus with loudness (independently of each other) was demonstrable to a similar extent when ratings on the nine-point loudness scale were used. Mean rating on the nine-point scale for those with tinnitus of ten or fewer years standing was 3.6 rising to 4 for those who had had tinnitus longer. Similarly those aged 60 or younger had nine-point scale means of 3.6 while older respondents had a mean scale value of 3.9. All in all, it would appear that tinnitus may be rated as being louder the longer the person has it or the older they are, but the differences are hardly a cause for worry or concern.

The above findings based upon all respondents in the survey were further analysed in an attempt to see what effect previous noise exposure appeared to have on whether tinnitus seemed to be louder the longer respondents had it or the older they were. First an examination was made of the replies of respondents who had had *no* experience of working where it was impossible to converse even by shouting, nor any experience when shouting had to be used because it was difficult to converse. Among respondents with no such noise exposure a weak association was evident indicating that irrespective of the respondent's age, tinnitus tended to be rated as (slightly) louder the longer that individuals had had it, and this was evident using both scales for measuring loudness ($P < 0.001$ adj.: $P < 0.002$ nine-point). For the same respondents the relation between age and tinnitus loudness, independently of the length of time they had had tinnitus, was less clear cut. On the nine-point loudness scale no association was evident that could not be explained by chance factors in the data, while the association on the adjectival scale data was more robust, only being likely to be due to chance in two instances in 100. For respondents with *no* experience of noisy work environments it would seem that tinnitus might appear slightly louder the longer they have had it, but whether or not tinnitus will appear louder due to age *per se* is not quite as evident. In any event the differences in loudness are of a degree not to cause individuals concern. What these results also illustrate is the difficulty of getting a reliable measure of loudness through a questionnaire.

For those respondents *with* some experience of work environments in which it was impossible to converse even by shouting, *none* of the previously mentioned associations were apparent and the same was true for respondents who had experience with work environments where it was difficult to converse. A final analysis was under-

117

taken on the data from respondents who had *no* experience of noisy work conditions, no experience of explosions or gun-fire, and who never went regularly to discos. Among this group of respondents the length of time they had had tinnitus *was* associated with its loudness, on both loudness measures (when age of respondent was controlled for; $P < 0.001$ adj.: $P < 0.004$ nine-point scale), although again the association was only mildly positive and the increase in loudness with the length of time the respondent had had tinnitus would not be of a degree to cause individuals worry. In this population of respondents exposed to the least noise, no significant association between age of respondent and loudness was observed (when length of time the respondent had had tinnitus was controlled for).

Overall, then, it would seem that the progression of tinnitus loudness from onset, or associated with current age of respondent, is likely to remain more constant among those who have experienced noisy environments than among those with no such experience. For respondents with no experience of noisy environments, tinnitus *may* appear louder in older age groups, but clearly not to the extent that it may appear louder the longer the person has had the tinnitus. In either case the extent of the change is slight, nothing to be worried about, and the likelihood of such a change for any individual, though there, is not strong.

DEVELOPMENT SINCE ONSET — THE CURRENT STUDY

Respondents in our study were asked — 'Can you describe the way in which the tinnitus has developed from the time it first started, on the lines below' and they were given three lines on which to write an open-ended answer. Some respondents may have thought that a question about the *development* of tinnitus implied describing *changes* in it, and having none, thought it inappropriate to answer the question. We believe this last reason is the most likely explanation for the generally low response.

Location

Of the 29 per cent of the overall sample who answered this question in terms of location, the vast majority — 69 per cent — said that the tinnitus had remained in the same location since onset, whatever that location happened to be. Twenty-five per cent reported that it had

118

developed in both ears since onset. A minuscule number reported odd changes: in one person it started in one ear but stopped in that ear and developed in the other; and in other cases the tinnitus moved from the ear or ears to some position within the head. For the vast majority of respondents it is likely that the tinnitus remained in the same location since onset. There may be about a seven in 100 chance that those with tinnitus starting in one ear may eventually develop tinnitus in the other as well.

Type of sound

Some 36 per cent of all respondents made mention of changes in the type of noise. However, 55 per cent of these respondents also spontaneously mentioned that the type of sound had remained the same. Just over 31 per cent mentioned that the sound had changed over time, but in such a multitude of diverse ways that no clear picture emerged of typical ways in which the type of sound had changed since onset. Over 13 per cent of respondents answering the question mentioned that a new sound had appeared, so that they had the original sound plus an additional sound (in some few cases respondents developed more than one additional sound). Placing these figures in the context of the overall sample of 984 respondents it would seem that for the great majority the type of sound will remain the same as it was at onset, but that for about one in ten respondents the type of sound might change in subtle and intricate ways (and in some few cases in dramatic ways). For some one in 20 respondents there is the likelihood that over time a new noise might appear in addition to the original one.

Change in loudness

Of the respondents mentioning this topic in reply to the open-ended question (some 56 per cent of the entire sample), 3.8 per cent mentioned that the tinnitus had got louder as they had got deafer, i.e. they associated these two events in their own minds; 5.4 per cent reported that the tinnitus had got *less* noticeable. One-third reported that the tinnitus had remained the same in loudness and 8.4 per cent mentioned variations in loudness that did not present any particularly systematic picture. Almost half of the respondents answering the question, however, said that the tinnitus had got more noticeable since onset. This indicates for the overall sample that between one in three and one in four respondents mentioned that the tinnitus had become more noticeable over time. But for the great majority of respondents, then, we may reasonably infer that the tinnitus seemed to have remained the same in loudness since onset.

Change in continuity

In response to the open-ended question about changes in the tinnitus since its onset, 34 per cent of the overall sample gave answers that concerned the continuity of the tinnitus. Of these respondents just under 60 per cent spontaneously mentioned that the tinnitus had remained the same. Between 5 and 6 per cent reported diverse changes in continuity that presented no clear picture, while 1.5 per cent reported that the tinnitus had become intermittent over time (whereas before, presumably, it had been more continuous). Nearly 4 per cent mentioned that bouts of tinnitus had become more frequent, and 3.6 per cent mentioned that bouts of tinnitus now lasted longer. Twenty-seven per cent of those whose tinnitus was not continuous at onset reported that it had developed into a continuous form.

The general picture of the development of tinnitus from onset for the great majority of respondents was that the tinnitus had remained the same. Tendencies to change were in the direction of the tinnitus becoming more noticeable and more continuous. Decreases in noticeability and continuity occurred, but were rare.

9

Psychological and Related Factors Influencing Tinnitus

WORRIES

Towards the end of our survey questionnaire respondents were asked the direct question — 'Does your tinnitus worry you?' Just under one-third of the sample suggested in one way or another that the tinnitus no longer worried them. The 'worries' that most predominated in the respondents' answers, in rank order of their occurrence, were: that there was no cure, relief or respite from the tinnitus (13 per cent); that it made them feel depressed (12.9 per cent); that it might get worse (10.4 per cent); that it was a perpetual irritation (10.3 per cent); that it spoiled their hearing (8.9 per cent); that it spoiled their social life (8.5 per cent); that it prevented concentration (7.7 per cent); that it prevented them having a rest or getting to sleep (5.7 per cent); and that it might lead to deafness (5 per cent).

That such worries may have taken their toll on individuals is perhaps best exemplified by Douek's remark about the *appearance* of his tinnitus patients — their appearance led him to usually overestimate their age by about ten years! (Coles, *et al.* 1981). Perhaps it is not too surprising that it is the 'no cure, no relief, no respite' element of tinnitus that for many people is the most frequently mentioned worry. Hallam *et al.* (1984) after comparing 20 'complaining' and 20 'non-complaining' patients showed that in both groups it was the 'persistence' of the tinnitus rather than either its loudness or its quality that was the main reason for its objectionable nature. Their conclusion, albeit based on small samples, was that complainers as opposed to non-complainers were more persistently aware of their noises, and found them more distracting at work.

The second most commonly mentioned worry in our sample was that tinnitus made the respondents depressed. Again this is intuitively not surprising: most people without tinnitus, but with some sensitivity, might well imagine that having a head noise all day, every day, with the likelihood that it would continue forever, was a depressing prospect. Several doctors responsible for running tinnitus clinics have remarked on the large extent of depression among tinnitus patients. The medical adviser to the British Tinnitus Association remarks that people with tinnitus are often depressed and that alleviation of the depression can often help them cope with the tinnitus. He suggests that up to half the patients reaching his tinnitus clinic may be depressed, many of whom might benefit from anti-depression therapy. Similarly, House (1981b) reports that many of the patients reaching her practice were very depressed and Wood, Webb, Orchick and Shea (1983) suggest that anxiety and depression are more common in people with tinnitus than in people in general or in people with other forms of hearing disorders. They also suggest that such levels of depression can build up to suicidal ideas in some individuals. In a study of 200 tinnitus patients Goodey reports that 20 per cent were 'frankly depressed', i.e. in definite need of treatment for depression, and 8 per cent were irritated by the tinnitus (House 1981c).

Having tinnitus must *make* many individuals depressed, but Hazell (in House 1981c) suggests that in half of his tinnitus-clinic patients with depression, there was a history of depressive illness *before* the tinnitus started, and that in those patients, once the tinnitus appeared it tended to be a 'welcome focus' for the patient's depression — i.e. it gave them something tangible to blame for their depression for which they themselves could not be held responsible.

Given that tinnitus does provide an only too clear focus, and may draw the individual's attention to the body and bodily functions, it is perhaps surprising to find that Goodey (in House 1981c) reports that in a comparison of pain sufferers and tinnitus sufferers there was much less evidence of hypochondria among those with tinnitus than among those with pain. It is clear that whether depression may herald tinnitus in some cases or whether tinnitus might herald depression in others, the depression itself and any anxiety should be treated.

Table 9.1 gives a more complete listing of the worries our respondents associated with their tinnitus.

One negative facet of tinnitus is the degree of 'annoyance' it can produce. Penner (1983) suggests that one element connected with the annoyance of tinnitus is its changeability. For eleven individuals with tinnitus and sensorineural hearing loss (loss due to damage in

Table 9.1: Worries associated with having tinnitus

Worry	Per cent
No cure, relief, respite	13.0
Causes depression	12.9
Tinnitus may get worse	10.4
An irritation	10.3
Spoils hearing	8.9
Affects social life	8.5
Prevents concentration	7.7
Prevents rest or sleep	5.7
May lead to deafness	5.0
Spoils hobbies, music	4.7
Can never enjoy silence	4.6
Makes work more difficult	4.1
Causes stress	3.5
Makes me think there's something wrong in my head	3.0
Causes tiredness	2.0
Makes me feel ill	1.2

Note: The percentage figures are based on 984 respondents, but many respondents gave more than one worry.
Source: The present study.

the cells that convert sound waves into nerve impulses, or damage in those nerves carrying the impulses onwards), Penner plotted the loudness of a 'shushing' (broad-band) noise needed to mask the tinnitus over a 30-minute period. The loudness of the noise required to mask the tinnitus grew, in some cases dramatically, over time, and the *annoyance* of the tinnitus (as reported on a five-point scale) related to the *rate* of change in the loudness of the masker, which presumably reflected a rate of change in the apparent loudness of the tinnitus. For these subjects Penner concluded that the *annoyance* of the tinnitus was governed by the *changes* in the tinnitus.

McFadden (1982) offers a speculative explanation as to why in many cases apparently low levels of tinnitus loudness, as objectively measured, seem to have little bearing on its annoyance level. Although one partial explanation for this apparent discrepancy between the loudness and the annoyance of the tinnitus is that the objective methods of loudness estimation simply *under-estimate* the loudness, McFadden considers that neural mechanisms in the brain may be attempting to make tinnitus conform to the 'rules' that govern the perception (and masking) of *external* noises. He cites evidence for tinnitus *not* behaving as if it were an external sound and suggests that:

. . . this and other aberrant behaviours 'bring the tinnitus to the attention' of certain neural mechanisms that persist in unsuccessful attempts to force the tinnitus to conform to the behaviour of external sounds and that their ongoing failure reaches consciousness as annoyance. (p. 47)

How accurate this suggestion is remains to be tested. It is clear, however, that a variety of factors appear to make tinnitus worse, more annoying, more noticeable or louder — more of a nuisance or of an irritation.

Time of day

Respondents were asked to use a seven-point scale — from least noticeable (1) to most noticeable (7) — to rate how noticeable the tinnitus was at seven different times of the day from early morning, just after waking up, through to late evening and during the night. Hazell (1981b) reports that 26 per cent of those with tinnitus whom he studied reported tinnitus to be worst on awakening, 29 per cent said it was worst in the evenings, only 3 per cent said it was worst in the afternoon, while 41 per cent said it stayed the same all the time. House (1981c) states that most of her patients reported tinnitus becoming more noticeable in the late afternoon. Twenty-one per cent of our respondents considered their tinnitus to be most notice-able first thing in the morning. This may be influenced by the tendency for tinnitus to seem loud after sleeping. Only 1.3 per cent of our respondents thought the tinnitus was most noticeable in the mid-morning, 2.1 per cent at mid-day, 2.7 per cent at mid-afternoon. Tinnitus was reported to be most noticeable for 9 per cent of our respondents in the early evening rising to 23 per cent of respondents who said it was most noticeable in the late evening. Twenty-one per cent of respondents said it was most noticeable during the night. Clearly from these results, then, tinnitus seems to be most noticeable in the late evening, during the night, and first thing in the morning. The last two times have in common the fact that sleep may have preceded them. Of sleeping *during the day* the medical adviser to the BTA notes that this seems to make tinnitus very much worse and 80 per cent of his patients report this to be the effect, although it is not clear just why this should happen. He reports that 'cat-naps' of only five minutes can, in some individuals, make the noises much worse.

When women respondents in our survey who were at paid work

and those who appeared to be housewives were compared in terms of how noticeable the tinnitus was *during the day*, clear (statistically significant) differences were obtained showing that housewives rated tinnitus as more noticeable during the day than did women in paid work. There were no such differences reported in the early morning, late evening, or during the night. Although the differences in noticeability reported during the day were not great in terms of degree, they were unlikely to have been due to chance. It may be the case that the environment of the housewife during the day, the home, is quieter on the whole than that of the woman at paid work, and that this makes the tinnitus more noticeable. But it may also be the case that, while appreciating that housewives *work* in the home, the nature of the work may, in general terms, be less attention-focusing than is that undertaken by women in paid employment.

SLEEP DIFFICULTIES

Hazell (1979b) reports that tinnitus rarely, if ever, wakes people once they are asleep, and the question 'Does the tinnitus ever wake you up?' might appear intuitively odd — if you are asleep you *are* asleep and, since while asleep you are, almost by definition, not conscious of the tinnitus, it seems at first glance odd to expect that anyone might attribute being woken up to the tinnitus. But individuals *do* attribute being woken up to *external* noises — to the spouse snoring or the baby crying, for example, so we were interested to see how many respondents in our study considered that the tinnitus woke them up. In response to our question 'Does the tinnitus ever wake you up?' 23.2 per cent of the entire sample said 'yes'. Furthermore, of those who said yes, 30 per cent reported that it happened every night!

Respondents were also asked 'Does the tinnitus give you any difficulty in getting to sleep?' Shailer, Tyler and Coles (1981), reporting some of the Institute of Hearing Research findings about the incidence of persistent tinnitus in the general population, note that about 6 per cent of their sample of some 7000 respondents indicated that tinnitus interfered with their getting to sleep. This sample will, of course, comprise a large proportion of individuals (maybe as many as 33 out of 34) with relatively mild tinnitus. In contrast Vernon (in Coles *et al.* 1981) notes that among his patients who complain of severe tinnitus and who are clinically judged to *have* severe tinnitus, 'only' about 50 per cent suffer from sleep

125

disturbances. Of the latter figure McFadden (1982) expresses surprise, suggesting that he would have thought sleep disturbance to have been even more common. In our sample just under 40 per cent of the respondents said 'yes' to the question 'Does the tinnitus give you any difficult in getting to sleep?' and of those saying 'yes' nearly 58 per cent said that this happened every night of the week. Those reporting difficulties in getting to sleep were significantly more likely also to be those reporting that the tinnitus had woken them up. There would appear, then, to be a substantial number of respondents in our overall sample, about one in five, for whom tinnitus makes it difficult every night of the week for them to get to sleep. Many of these individuals are those who feel they are also woken up regularly by the tinnitus and who consequently may be particularly debilitated and tired.

Among our sample, tinnitus loudness (as measured on both the nine-point and the adjectival scales) was significantly associated with difficulties the respondents had in getting to sleep ($r = 0.248$, $P < 0.001$) — the louder the tinnitus the more nights a week the respondent was likely to say he or she had such difficulties. This relation remained significant when the possible effects of the respondents' (self-estimated) hearing acuity were taken into account ($r = 0.321$, $P < 0.001$), although when the influence of tinnitus loudness was removed it appeared that *better* hearing was significantly associated with increased sleep problems ($r = 0.119$, $P < 0.001$). A variety of other analyses demonstrated that louder-rated tinnitus was associated with increasing number of nights a week that respondents experienced difficulty getting to sleep. Meikle and Taylor-Walsh (1984), reporting results from a study of over 1800 tinnitus clinic patients, also noted that reported severity of tinnitus and sleep disturbance are strongly associated. In our study an examination of the rated loudness of the tinnitus with whether respondents reported being *woken up* by the tinnitus showed that louder tinnitus was significantly associated with this form of sleep disturbance. Coles (1984a), however, counsels that sleep disturbance alone should not be taken as a clinical indicator of severity, since some individuals with severe tinnitus may *not* have sleep problems. He also notes (1984b) that women are more likely to report sleep disturbances due to tinnitus than are men. This finding was reproduced in our study both in terms of difficulties in getting to sleep and in being woken up by the tinnitus ($P < 0.001$).

126

PERSONALITY FACTORS

In terms of *reacting* to tinnitus, it is likely that individuals who are more inward-looking than outward-looking, shy than gregarious (more introverted than extroverted), may be more likely to take notice of the tinnitus and hence report annoyance from it. Hallam *et al.* (1984) reported that both tinnitus 'complainers' and tinnitus 'non-complainers' were slightly introverted, a result that agreed with Green's (1976) finding that introversion rather than neuroticism (as evidenced in counter-productive behaviour patterns, often of an obsessional type, that are recognised as such by the neurotic individual) distinguished his tinnitus group from the general population, although Green did find that among his sample increased neuroticism was associated with increased *annoyance* from the tinnitus. Introverts *may* spend more time in relatively quiet surroundings and present themselves with more opportunity to listen to tinnitus and, once it is perceived, may be slightly more likely than extroverts to dwell on this internal phenomenon. Those individuals who *do* have neurotic obsessional tendencies may find that tinnitus presents a very tangible thing to get obsessed about. As House (1981c) points out when talking about the personality of the tinnitus patient:

> Tinnitus as a symptom can become a scapegoat. Conflicts and needs are displaced on this symptom; it can be a chief concern and often an obsession. This obsession leads to other neurotic behaviour such as social withdrawal, isolation and difficulty with reality contact. In some cases the tinnitus seems to take on the role of secondary gain; it can relieve the guilt associated with job failure or social conflicts, for example. (p. 198)

Wood *et al.* (1983) also notes that there does appear to be a group of tinnitus complainers who cling to the symptoms for psychological support and who resist any treatment techniques despite their complaints.

Hallam *et al.* (1984) note the not uncommonly reported 'fact' that tinnitus has led to a change of personality — usually in terms of increased irritability, and it may be remembered that just under 3 per cent of our sample of respondents reported being worried because the tinnitus had made them more irritable. Certainly anecdotal evidence from the first author's local self-help group suggests that 'increased irritability' is the 'personality change' most readily observed by both the 'sufferer' and his or her spouse and close relatives. Further psychological consequences of having tinnitus will depend on the individual's predispositions and sensitivities.

HEADACHES AND EAR DISCOMFORT

One common effect of tinnitus, sheerly as a bodily symptom, is that it is associated with headaches. The medical adviser to the BTA, in reply to a reader's letter, suggests that head pain from tinnitus is very common and that the vast majority of 'sufferers' have a lot of pain as a result of tension in the muscles of the neck, which causes headaches. He adds that pain often appears localised over the spot where the tinnitus seems loudest.

In our study, 35 per cent of respondents said they often got headaches, and one-third of these reported getting headaches at least twice a week. Overall, one in every 100 of our respondents reported getting a headache every day. The number of headaches experienced was significantly related to the loudness of tinnitus, those with louder tinnitus being more prone to headaches ($P < 0.001$). Another bodily symptom associated with tinnitus can be pain or discomfort in the ear. Forty-two per cent of our respondents said they sometimes got pain and discomfort, 5.4 per cent said they often did, and 1.5 per cent said they had pain and discomfort in their ears all the time. Such pain and discomfort was significantly more likely than expected, on a chance basis, to be reported by respondents who rated their tinnitus as loud ($P < 0.001$) and by those who reported getting changes in the pitch of their tinnitus ($P < 0.001$).

Ear pain or discomfort was also, as expected, associated with the tinnitus location, usually being at or near the ear with the tinnitus (in those respondents whose tinnitus appeared localised at the ears). One might infer that subjectively louder forms of tinnitus *a priori* might be expected to be more stressful (although complaint behaviour and symptom severity have not been shown to be necessarily strongly associated). Obviously, headaches and forms of ear pain and discomfort are themselves stressful. The extent to which the individual can cope with these forms of stress will be largely dependent on the other stresses in his or her life, as well as his or her own psychological characteristics. That there is a psychosomatic interaction is suggested by the observation that variation in reported distress from tinnitus is often in synchrony with other life stresses such as, for example, physical illnesses, redundancy or threat of prosecution (Hallam *et al.* 1984). Given the 'fact' of tinnitus as a *bodily* symptom, and the other bodily symptoms that may be associated with it, it is perhaps not too surprising to find House (1981c) reporting that patients come to see their disorder as physical in nature — which it is — and many of them resist a 'psychological interpretation' in the first stages of treatment. McFadden (1982, pp. 56–57) nicely sums up the situation with regard to psychological factors in tinnitus, as follows:

> . . . it is imperative to realise that the plight of tinnitus sufferers has, until very recently, been largely ignored, and, as a consequence the discovery of variations from the 'normal' in their psychological profiles cannot be unequivocally identified as cause or effect of their tinnitus problem . . . This is not to say that, once present, a tinnitus will not be better handled by one person than another, nor that transient psychological difficulties cannot cause people to focus on, or exaggerate, a pre-existing or new physiological malady; the point is that psychological makeup is probably a minor *contributing* factor to the underlying anomaly . . .
>
> The temptation is often great to refer such cases to psychotherapists; in the past this course has often been pursued too hastily — and ineffectively — since many patients balk at such treatment for what they strongly regard to be a physiological problem.

Although individuals' capacities to deal with stress *do* vary, for several different reasons, it is clear that the noticeability of tinnitus *is* related to stress and mood-tone.

STRESS, ANXIETY, DEPRESSION, FATIGUE AND MOOD-TONE

Respondents in our survey were asked to note if there was any change in the noticeability of tinnitus depending on their mood. Respondents could indicate that there was no change, that the tinnitus was more noticeable, or that it appeared less noticeable. One item related to fatigue — tiredness — two items related to stress and tension, and the remaining five items referred to mood-tone — when sad, angry, relaxed, happy and depressed.

Noticeability when tired

House (1981c) comments that most of her patients reported that the noise became more noticeable when they felt tired. Elsewhere House (1981b) noted that almost all patients reported their head noise was worse with fatigue (and conflict). Seventy per cent of our respondents indicated that the noticeability of the tinnitus changed for the worse, i.e. became more noticeable, when they were tired. Twenty seven per cent reported no change and only 2.6 per cent indicated that the tinnitus was less noticeable when they were tired. Clearly, then, among our respondents, tiredness and tinnitus noticeability go more or less hand in glove.

Noticeability when relaxed and when happy

Forty-two per cent of our respondents answering the item about 'when happy' reported that the tinnitus was less noticeable when they were happy; 55.5 per cent reported no change in noticeability; and 2.6 per cent said the tinnitus was more noticeable when they were happy. Clearly, then, only in a very few individuals does tinnitus become more noticeable when the person is happy. Similarly, only 11. 9 per cent of respondents replying to the item 'when relaxed' said the tinnitus was more noticeable; 52.1 per cent reported no change; and 36 per cent said the tinnitus was less noticeable.

Noticeability when sad and when depressed

Sadness and depression are not identical, but they intuitively have overtones of dejectedness and despondency, of feeling 'low' and miserable. Thirty per cent of those responding to the item 'when sad' reported that the tinnitus was more noticeable; 67 per cent reported 'no change'; and only 2.4 per cent said the tinnitus was less noticeable when they were sad. Over 57 per cent reported that the tinnitus was more noticeable when depressed, with 41.3 per cent reporting 'no change' and only 1 per cent saying the tinnitus was less noticeable when they were depressed. Clearly, then, sadness and depression are not associated with a lessening in the noticeability of tinnitus.

Noticeability when angry

Over 9 per cent of those replying to the item 'when angry' reported that the tinnitus was less noticeable; 51.1 per cent reported that it remained the same; and 39.3 per cent reported that the tinnitus was more noticeable when they were angry. Graham (1981c) reported that eight of the 46 hearing-impaired children with tinnitus whom he studied said that tinnitus tended to appear when they were tense or angry.

Noticeability when under stress or when tense

People who report they are under stress may not necessarily report feeling tense, and vice versa, but tension is often a consequence of periods of stress, and perceived bodily tension is often attributed to stress. Given the juxtaposition of the two, it is perhaps not too surprising to find an almost identical response pattern to these two items. About two-thirds of those responding to 'when tense' and 'when under stress' indicated that the tinnitus was more noticeable, and under one-third reported 'no change'; the remaining few reported that the tinnitus was less noticeable when they were tense or under stress. Hazell (1979c) considers that 'virtually everyone' with tinnitus will say that it is much worse when they are under stress.

10

Non-medically Related Factors Influencing Tinnitus

There are as yet no published systematic studies of the influence of dietary factors on the production or annoyance characteristics of tinnitus — but anecdotal evidence suggests that for some individuals dietary factors certainly *do* play a role. Goodey (1981) goes as far as saying that it seems that almost *any* material ingested or inhaled into the body can cause or aggravate tinnitus in particular cases. Unfortunately, the fact that some food seems to exacerbate tinnitus in some individuals may be irrelevant to the vast majority of those with tinnitus. In our sample, 25 per cent of respondents with answers codable under the 'tinnitus is worse when . . .' category mentioned food and drink, which would be an absolute minimum of 3 per cent of our overall sample. The medical adviser to the BTA suggests that in about 10 per cent of sufferers the tinnitus is exacerbated by things in their diet. In some cases the exacerbation may be more due to the mechanics of jaw movement in eating certain foods (crunchy peanuts, for example), than to the food itself. Readers' letters to the British Tinnitus Association often raise the question about the influence of foods, and some readers offer diets that seem to have made them 'tinnitus-free'. In many instances individuals may have mild allergies or sensitivities to certain foods, illustrated dramatically during part of the general discussion at the end of the Ciba Symposium on Tinnitus:

> **Dr. Tonndorf:** Certain foods are believed to trigger off tinnitus. For example, when Dr. E.L. Derlacki of Chicago eats strawberries he experiences full-scale Menière's symptoms, including tinnitus.
> **Dr. J.W. House:** We are really talking about allergies here, and tinnitus in these cases is probably related to endolymphatic

hydrops [part of the Menière's syndrome], which can be mediated through allergies. The treatment we provide for such patients is largely a question of controlling their hydrops, rather than their tinnitus. (Evered and Lawrenson, 1981, p. 234)

Later in the discussion Goodey remarks that in taking case-histories from patients with intermittent tinnitus, his team occasionally find there is a dietary-related tinnitus — and he mentions orange cordials in this context. If dietary factors are suspected, a 'screening procedure' is used in which the individual is put on a 'caveman' diet of a limited range of fruit and vegetables and lean meat for ten days. If the individual has ten days free from the tinnitus symptoms, the treatment is pursued further to detect what dietary elements may be responsible. Elsewhere Goodey (1981) reports that in his experience the foods most commonly identified as a cause of tinnitus have been cheese and chocolate.

Prompted by a suggestion from a local Professor of Biology whose tinnitus appeared to become consistently more noticeable after a heavy meal, we asked our respondents if they experienced the same effect. Only 10.8 per cent of respondents said there was some change in the tinnitus after a heavy meal, and of these three-quarters said it became *more* noticeable, while 17.5 per cent said it became *less* noticeable and 7.9 per cent reported that the tinnitus changed to a pulsatile form. Responses to the question may have been partially influenced by the circumstances in which heavy meals might be taken — at the end of the day, on special occasions, in company and so forth. It may be the case, however, that in some individuals the change in blood flow through the micro-structure of the ear that could occur as blood is directed to increased activity in the digestive system has some influence on tinnitus loudness or noticeability. Thirteen respondents spontaneously wrote that although the tinnitus did not appear to change with a heavy meal alone, it *did* change when the heavy meal was accompanied by alcohol — in 11 instances getting more noticeable.

These apparently idiosyncratic responses to the ingestion of food, while indicative of the complexity of the factors that impinge on tinnitus noticeability, should not be taken to suggest that individuals with tinnitus should obsessively monitor the influence of their diet. However, an increased awareness of the possibility that dietary factors may play a part may help some individuals see a connection between their own diet and tinnitus noticeability that they had not thought of before. Government legislation resulting in the publicising of food additives has surprised, if not shocked, many people at the numbers of chemicals that are added to what they had taken to be 'good, wholesome food'. Some individuals may find it adds variety to their life, if in the event little else, to change to an 'additive free' health food diet for a while to see if it has any effect on their tinnitus. Pulec, Hodell and Anthony (1978) suggest that reduction to an ideal weight and control of serum cholesterol (by cutting down on the intake of animal fats), can reduce tinnitus in some of those individuals who may have 'ear allergies' due to food.

DRINK

Caffeine

There is some general anecdotal evidence that the main culprit exacerbating tinnitus for some individuals as far as drink is concerned is coffee — the caffeinated variety. Both the medical adviser to the British Tinnitus Association and Goodey (1981) suggest that it is worthwhile cutting strong coffee out of one's diet to see if this has any effect. Goodey also suggests that strong tea may exacerbate tinnitus in some individuals. The caffeine in coffee and tea stimulates the nervous system and has various effects upon blood pressure and blood vessels, widening blood vessels in the skin, and narrowing those that supply the brain — it is a 'pick-me-up' that activates the brain and helps people to think clearly. The exact mechanism by which caffeine may influence tinnitus in some people is not known, but since caffeine leads to stimulation rather than relaxation, the effect might be psychological as well as physiological. Caffeine is not only an ingredient of tea and coffee, colas usually contain caffeine, as does cocoa. It is also present in numerous over-the-counter tonics and pain relievers. The average caffeine content of a cup of tea is 50 to 100 mg, and of coffee is 100 to 200 mg. In many people a dose of 100 mg will produce adverse effects, such as difficulty in sleeping, restlessness, excitement and trembling — and ringing in the ears. It is not too arduous a task to avoid taking caffeine-containing products to see if this has any effect on the noticeability of tinnitus. Products containing quinine for example, tonic water, should be avoided for similar reasons. In the treatment of malaria, after prolonged high doses, quinine will induce tinnitus, but some individuals may be particularly susceptible to its effect in small doses.

Alcohol

Alcohol is often wrongly thought to be a stimulant but it is in fact a sedative and has the effect of widening the blood vessels, which in the micro-structure of the blood supply to the ear may influence the tinnitus. Nicotinic acid — not to be confused with nicotine — has a similar effect. Alcohol may have little or no effect on tinnitus among many individuals, but may appear to make it 'worse' in some and 'better' in others. It has been suggested that 5 per cent of tinnitus sufferers find alcohol makes the tinnitus worse and Spitzer (1981) notes that alcohol has long been regarded as an ear-damaging (ototoxic) agent resulting in tinnitus when used in excess. Even the Romans in 30 AD were advised to stop drinking wine as a means of reducing tinnitus (Stephens 1984). Goodey (1981, p. 268) points out that excess alcohol can induce tinnitus in almost anyone and certain alcoholic drinks can induce it in susceptible individuals. One reader of the BTA Newsletter reports being tinnitus-free for three months after stopping drinking gin in the evening, but unfortunately after three months the tinnitus returned. There might not, of course, have been any real connection between the two events. Goodey (1981) suggests that in his experience red wine, and grain-based spirits such as whisky and bourbon and some gins and vodkas are the commonest forms of alcohol to produce tinnitus. Alcohol for some individuals does seem to produce a *lessening* in the noticeability of tinnitus, although McFadden (1982) suggests that this may be more due to its apparent psychologically relaxing qualities than to a direct effect on the cause of tinnitus. In a study of 57 tinnitus sufferers who were 'alcohol users', Ronis (1984) reports that nine considered it made the tinnitus better and four considered it made the tinnitus worse. However, it was those most likely to be suffering damage through high levels of alcohol consumption who reported most relief.

SMOKING

All the currently available evidence that relates to smoking — be it of tobacco or marijuana — and tinnitus is largely anecdotal.

135

Tobacco

The main drug in tobacco is nicotine. Small doses stimulate nerve-endings in both the sympathetic ('readiness'-inducing) and parasympathetic ('calmness'-inducing) parts of the autonomic nervous system (that not under conscious control). One of these effects is constriction or narrowing of the blood vessels. In habitual smokers sympathetic reflexes predominate, with raised blood pressure being one effect. It is possible that in individuals reporting effects due to tobacco smoking it is blood pressure and supply factors that play a role. Both Schleuning (1981) and Tyler (in Evered and Lawrenson 1981, p. 235) suggest that smoking may exacerbate tinnitus in certain individuals, and McFadden (1982) mentions that Fowler (1942) asserted smoking to be a common cause of tinnitus. Fowler also suggested that it was necessary to give up smoking for at least one month in order to eliminate it as a causative factor. Study of this area is fraught with problems. Habitual smokers on a non-smoking regimen are likely to be suffering withdrawal symptoms — to be feeling tense and irritable, 'on edge'. In such a state the tinnitus might appear more noticeable, hence the need to ensure such reactions can be eliminated when examining the effects of smoking on tinnitus.

Among our respondents, smokers on a variety of analyses were significantly more likely to rate their tinnitus as louder (on both loudness scales) than non-smokers ($P < 0.001$). Some of those with louder forms of tinnitus may smoke to 'calm their nerves' because of the tinnitus, but in some of these smokers the act of smoking may well be exacerbating the noticeability of the tinnitus or actually making it louder. Interestingly, those smokers who had been smoking for 38 or more years reported a quieter tinnitus (on the nine-point loudness scale but not on the adjectival loudness scale) than did those who had been smoking for 37 years or less ($t = 1.14$, $df = 219$, $P = 0.011$). They also reported the tinnitus to be less noticeable first thing in the morning and in the late evening ($t = 2.15$, $df = 205$, $P = 0.03$; $t = 2.01$, $df = 202$, $P = 0.045$) but more noticeable at midday ($t = 1.98$, $df = 191$, $P = 0.049$) than did smokers who had been smoking for 37 years or less. No such differences in loudness or variations in noticeability throughout the day were found between inhalers and non-inhalers.

Marijuana

Schleuning (1981) considers that marijuana has frequently been an exacerbator of tinnitus and reports having five patients with a neuro-sensory hearing loss that he links to their heavy use of the drug. Vernon (in Evered and Lawrenson 1981, p. 168) reports details of 17 patients attending his clinic who were musicians, and who had a noise-induced hearing loss plus a noise-induced tinnitus. All 17 had been taking marijuana and they reported about a five-fold increase in the tinnitus after using the drug. Vernon notes that this may be either because their attention is focused more closely on the tinnitus or because their tinnitus actually becomes louder, and points out the need for objective measures of tinnitus loudness so that attentional effects can be separated from real changes in tinnitus quality.

Smokers may feel that going without cigarettes for at least one month is a high price to have to pay to find out if smoking is exacerbating their tinnitus. On the other hand, the potential disappointment of finding out that it is *not* so affected, may be counterbalanced by the fact that the smoker may by that time be well on the road to being a non-smoker — which can only be to his or her advantage, irrespective of the tinnitus.

EXACERBATION OF TINNITUS BY NOISE

Respondents in our survey were asked — 'Are there any sounds which make the tinnitus more noticeable *when they are present*?' Twenty-eight per cent of respondents replied that there were such sounds. Two blank lines were provided to enable respondents to describe the sounds that when present made the tinnitus more noticeable. Table 10.1 gives a detailed breakdown of how the respondents' replies were classified.

Clearly Table 10.1 demonstrates that a variety of loud sounds or noises were predominantly responsible for making the tinnitus more noticeable when they were present. A second group of sounds with the same effect seem to be those characterised by a high pitch. Over 12 per cent of respondents from the entire sample, i.e. one in eight respondents, mentioned one sound that made the tinnitus more noticeable; 6.1 per cent mentioned two; 2.6 per cent mentioned three; 2.1 per cent mentioned four; and one individual listed eight different sorts of sounds or noises each of which made her tinnitus more noticeable.

137

Table 10.1 Sounds present that make tinnitus more noticeable

Sounds	Per cent[a]	
Loud machines	29.4	
Other loud sounds	14.5	
Sharp, sudden sounds	3.3	
Loud music	25.5	
A noisy environment	16.5	
Any loud noise	6.6	
High continuous noises	10.6	
Other high-pitched noises	7.8	
High-pitched sounds	6.2	
TV or radio	10.2	
Hammering	2.3	
Quiet sounds	4.3	
Playing a musical instrument	2.3	(Base = 255 respondents)

Note: a. Respondents could list as many such noises as was appropriate.
Source: The present study.

Respondents were then asked if there were any sounds that made the tinnitus more noticeable when the sound had just finished (e.g. after a loud bang). Twenty-seven per cent of the overall sample said that there were such sounds, and these are detailed in Table 10.2.

Again it is clear from Table 10.2 that loud sounds predominate in making tinnitus more noticeable. However, more respondents reported the influence of sudden sharp sounds, and hammering, as making tinnitus more noticeable when they had *finished*, than when they were *present*. This may have been partly due to the fact that 'a loud bang' was used as an example in the question itself.

Clearly a significant number of our respondents considered that their tinnitus was affected by loud sounds, and the first author can make his tinnitus jump in loudness for a fraction of a second by clapping his hands near his ears. Hallam *et al.* (1984) reported that, among their subjects, tinnitus in *both* ears was more likely to be associated with tinnitus being made worse by noise, and 43 per cent of their subjects considered to have a noise-induced hearing loss reported that the tinnitus was made worse by noise, as against 15 per cent of patients whose hearing loss was not thought to be noise induced. We could not replicate from the data from our respondents the Hallam *et al.* findings about bilaterality of tinnitus (i.e. tinnitus in both ears) and its association with noise making tinnitus worse. A variety of analyses examining the effects of noise with regard to the location of the tinnitus showed no significant differences. However, those in our sample who had worked where it was impossible

Table 10.2: Sounds that when finished make tinnitus more noticeable

Sounds	Per cent[a]	
Loud machines	44.7	
Other loud noises	10.9	
Sharp, sudden sounds	26.7	
Loud music	15.3	
A noisy environment	15.3	
Any loud noise	7.0	
High continuous noises	3.5	
Other high-pitched noises	7.9	
High-pitched sounds	1.8	
TV or radio	2.2	
Hammering	4.8	
Quiet sounds	0	
Playing a musical instrument	0.8	(Base = 228 respondents)

Note: a. Respondents could list as many such noises as was appropriate.
Source: The present study.

or difficult to *converse* were significantly more likely to report that noises when present, or when finished made the tinnitus more noticeable ($P < 0.02$) although this did not appear to be affected by the length of time they had worked in such settings.

Individuals with tinnitus often feel that the tinnitus itself affects the intelligibility of speech. Forty-one per cent of our respondents replied 'yes' to the question 'Are you aware of the *tinnitus* making it difficult for you to hear speech?' Those with louder rated forms of tinnitus (on both loudness scales) were, on a variety of analyses, significantly more likely to say the tinnitus made it difficult for them to hear speech ($P < 0.0001$), as were those who had not got good hearing (self-assessed) in both ears ($P < 0.0001$). We may infer that respondents with loud tinnitus who also have hearing impairments will be those with particular difficulty hearing speech intelligibly.

EXACERBATION ON LYING DOWN

One specific question that respondents had been asked earlier in the questionnaire was 'Is there any noticeable change in the tinnitus when you lie down after you have been standing up?' The phrase 'after you have been standing up' was inserted to emphasise the change in body posture involved in lying down, although it is possible that replies to this question will be influenced by other factors, for example, most people may only lie down when they are in bed trying to get to sleep. One quarter of all respondents noticed changes that may at least be partially attributable to the physical act of lying down. For two-thirds of these respondents the tinnitus became more noticeable, for 20 per cent it became less noticeable, for 7 per cent the tinnitus changed in form to one that was more obviously pulsating in character, and 3 per cent of respondents mentioned various other changes of which one characteristic was a louder tinnitus. Clearly from these data, for a substantial majority of individuals, tinnitus seems more noticeable when they lie down (although, as noted earlier, this might be influenced by 'late at night' and 'tiredness' factors that we will discuss separately below).

Two of the hearing-impaired children in Graham's (1981c) study mentioned that they noticed their tinnitus came on when they lay down, and — the effects of quiet surroundings, time of day and tiredness apart — it would appear that for some individuals body posture may influence tinnitus.

In a previous chapter in the context of spontaneous noise emissions from the ear, we noted Wilson's (1980b) finding that in an inverted body position a continuous objective tone could be heard in one individual. Wilson and Sutton (1981) suggest that body posture determines the differences in height between the heart and the inner ear and thus influences the hydrostatic (fluid) pressure on the footplate of the third bone in the middle ear (the stapes footplate). Displacing this footplate would stretch and stiffen the fibrous bands (the annular ligament) that hold the footplate to the opening of the inner ear (the oval window), and might have a bearing on the production of some forms of mainly tonal tinnitus. The medical adviser to the BTA in reply to a reader's question about why the tinnitus seems worse on lying down noted that there is a change in fluid pressure in the inner ear on lying down that may affect tinnitus. He suggested that the respondent use two or three pillows in order to try sleeping in a more upright position. McFadden (1982) considers that the recurrence of anecdotes about air-pressure changes and tinnitus reduction imply that mechanical attempts to relieve tinnitus, i.e. direct attempts to manipulate such pressure changes, may deserve greater attention for the purpose both of diagnosis and of treatment.

MISCELLANEOUS FACTORS ASSOCIATED WITH THE PRODUCTION OR EXACERBATION OF TINNITUS

Flying

It is often reported by tinnitus sufferers when as passengers on an aircraft, that when the plane comes in to land, it seems to exacerbate their tinnitus. This is largely due to the fact that changes in aircraft pressure may, particularly in individuals who have colds, lead to decreased pressure in the middle ear. This the eustachian tube may be unable to relieve because it does not open to allow air to pass from the nose to the middle ear; this happens to some individuals especially if the increase in cabin pressure on descending is sudden rather than gradual. The consequence is a temporary form of *conductive* deafness which means that external masking noises are lessened and the tinnitus thus appears louder or more clear. Swallowing for a while, which is usually accompanied by the opening of the eustachian tube, should help, otherwise pinching the nose while gently blowing into it with the mouth closed (the valsalva manoeuvre) should help equalise pressure between the middle ear and the outside (Hazell 1983).

Menstruation

It is possible that some women experience an exacerbation of tinnitus during menstruation; this is probably related to increased fluid retention at that time, which may affect fluid pressure in the inner ear. Just over one-quarter of our female respondents currently having regular periods reported that the tinnitus changed during the menstrual cycle, and nearly all such changes were in the direction of the tinnitus being more noticeable and one respondent said the tinnitus was much worse. Some respondents said that the tinnitus became more noticeable in the few days before a period started. *Pregnancy* seemed to have had a less clear-cut effect on those of our respondents who had tinnitus while pregnant, although those few who noticed a change (some 17 per cent) tended to report that the tinnitus was more noticeable.

Headaches

We have pointed out previously that many individuals get tension headaches in association with their tinnitus. House (1981a) suggests there may be a reflex arc, a nerve chain whose messages are not under conscious control, by which muscle tension in the face and neck seems to cause an apparent increase in tinnitus. It may be possible that headaches serve to focus attention even more closely on the head and the tinnitus. Those seeking to remedy headaches by medicines are best advised to avoid those that are aspirin-based and to use paracetamol instead.

Eye musculature and tinnitus

Conditioned reflexes may partly explain why some individuals seem to get tinnitus, or have their tinnitus exacerbated, in association with certain eye or eyelid movements. When Pavlov rang a bell at the same time as presenting hungry dogs with food he was eventually able to get the dogs to salivate to the bell irrespective of the presence of food. In a similar fashion nerve networks can evolve that produce an end product (in this example, salivation) in response to a 'peculiar' stimulus (in this case, a bell). Collard, Wagner and Tingwald (1982) report the case of a woman whose periodic 'rushing' tinnitus became extremely annoying whenever she tried to relax quietly. It was suggested that the woman had learned to bring her middle-ear muscles under conscious control as a means of relieving a perceived pressure in the ear. She had been blinking while doing this, and eventually the tinnitus, thought to be produced because of the contractions of the middle-ear muscles, was produced by eye-blinks. Each time she blinked she heard the 'rushing' noises. Williams (1980) reports the case of a 34-year-old man who had a three-year history of left-sided tinnitus when he blinked his eyes, and Whittaker (1982) reports the case of a woman who would get a monotone tinnitus in her right ear that diminished in loudness to nothing in two or three seconds when she squeezed her eyelids shut tightly or when she turned her eyes to the right. Whittaker (1983) reports the case of a man who noticed that his tinnitus abruptly increased in loudness for a period of five seconds or so, without any change in pitch, when he turned his eyes. Marchiando, Per-Lee and Jackson (1983) also mention patients who had subjective tinnitus that was synchronous with eyelid movements. No real explanation exists for these findings but they do illustrate how idiosynchratic the causation and exacerbation of tinnitus can be.

11

Medically Related Factors
Influencing Tinnitus

Shulman (1981a) refers to two earlier works, one of which suggested there were at least 22 known causes of tinnitus, and the other which took 15 pages to enumerate possible clinical causes. It is not too remarkable, then, to find Evans (1981b) in his chairman's closing comments at the Ciba Symposium on Tinnitus saying, a little ironically — 'To my surprise, at least, we have identified two conditions with which tinnitus is apparently *not* associated, i.e. hearing loss due to mumps and barbiturate poisoning!' The irony is there because he has begun to wonder if there isn't anything that *doesn't* cause tinnitus, at least in certain individuals.

Because tinnitus *is* so common, with 1 in 200 individuals in the general population experiencing considerable distress from tinnitus, it is only to be expected that in any subpopulation with other quite specific ailments, say rheumatism sufferers, the same incidence of tinnitus will obtain. No doubt in certain susceptible individuals various illnesses and diseases *do* bring on or exacerbate tinnitus, for reasons not yet known, which would not affect less susceptible individuals. For the vast majority the link between any present ailment and onset of tinnitus is likely to be statistically determined by the general prevalence of tinnitus.

MENIÈRE'S DISEASE

Hazell (1982a) reports that Menière's Disease affects 46 in every 100,000 persons in the general population and tends to be commoner in men than women. Its episodic symptoms are a spinning dizziness — the room or external environment feels to be turning round, and loss of hearing, which usually affects the low rather than the high frequencies, and which gets progressively worse, and tinnitus. The attacks are brought on unpredictably and the course of the disease in any one individual is also unpredictable. This means that it is often difficult to know if treatment by drugs, for example, is being effective, or whether the disease is in a period of remission.

Vernon, Johnson, and Schleuning (1980) consider that tinnitus in Menière's Disease is characteristically a low-pitched narrow band of noise usually described as a 'roaring sound' or a 'buzzing'. Tinnitus in Menière's Disease is often very easily masked by a suitable tinnitus masker and often by a hearing aid alone.

THYROID DISORDERS

An under-functioning thyroid (hypothyroidism) or an over-functioning thyroid (hyperthyroidism — and thyrotoxicosis) has been connected with the production of tinnitus as a symptom. Over functioning leads to increased fuel consumption by the body, irritability and restlessness, and loss of weight. Under functioning leads to myxoedema, often characterised by loss of energy, appetite and a dulled mind. Various specialists, cited by McFadden (1982), have suggested that screening for thyroid disorders should take place in tinnitus clinics.

DIABETES

In diabetes there is a shortage of insulin, which results in glucose not being taken up as fuel by the cells of the body; instead, the glucose accumulates in the blood. Fat combustion follows to provide fuel but is incomplete and leads to intermediate products — ketone bodies — which can be poisonous in sufficient quantities. Schleuning (1981) notes that diabetics for some reason have a much higher average incidence of tinnitus than 'normal' people and reports seeing a large percentage of patients with diabetes at his tinnitus clinic. Meyerhoff and Shrewsbury (1980) suggest that screening for diabetes should be routine when undertaking a thorough medical examination of the patient with tinnitus, as should tests for hypoglycaemia, a condition where there is a *deficiency* of sugar in the blood. This is usually caused by the presence of too much insulin, the consequence being that the brain gets starved of the fuel — glucose — that it needs.

CERVICAL SPONDYLOSIS

This is a condition in which there is a degenerative process or osteoarthritis of the upper segments of the backbone. In the neck this causes pressure on the nerve roots that emerge between vertebrae. Donaldson (1981) mentions cervical spine disease as a cause of tinnitus in some instances.

ARTHRITIS

Arthritis (inflammation of the tissues of one or more joints usually accompanied by pain and swelling) in the neck may possibly play some part in tinnitus. Care should be taken that the drugs prescribed for the relief of arthritis do not themselves exacerbate the tinnitus.

MULTIPLE OR DISSEMINATED SCLEROSIS

This is a chronic disease of the central nervous system in which small scattered areas of the brain and spinal cord degenerate and nerve fibres lose their insulating myelin sheaths and thus their ability to conduct electrical nerve impulses. Both Hazell (1979b) and McFadden (1982) suggest that just occasionally patients present with tinnitus as a symptom of such systemic diseases as multiple sclerosis. Tinnitus may also occasionally be a symptom in Paget's disease, in which the normal process of absorption and renewal of bones becomes disturbed and uncoordinated. Calcium loss leads to structural weakness and deformity, and later too much calcium is deposited and the bones are thickened. The disease can effect any bones, but in tinnitus production is most likely to affect those bones in close proximity to the hearing mechanism. Hazell (1979b) notes this as a possibility.

ZINC DEFICIENCY

Hazell (1984a), reporting papers presented at the Second International Tinnitus Seminar held in New York in 1983, mentions that there was much additional discussion about the drug therapies that have enjoyed some popularity in the United States, such as the use of zinc. Zinc deficiency can lead to anaemia, and Hazell considers

145

it likely that zinc treatment may be effective in patients who have a low blood level of zinc.

ANAEMIA

Anaemia is due to a shortage of oxygen-carrying pigment (haemoglobin) in the red blood cells. It may be caused by iron deficiency (sometimes due to bleeding into the stomach). Pernicious anaemia is caused by shortage of vitamin B12. In either form tinnitus might arise as a symptom (Donaldson 1981).

SYPHILIS

This sexually transmitted disease is caused by a bacterium that is part of the spirochaete family. In its third stage, which may occur after a dormant period of from two to ten years or longer during which no symptoms have been evident, the disease may begin to attack the nervous system and mucous membranes, among other things. Goodhill (1981) points out that the tinnitus might arise because the disease produces leaks between the various hitherto separate fluid systems in the inner ear and head.

COLDS AND CATARRH

Wilson and Sutton (1981) point out that a cold may produce reduction in pressure in the middle ear and this may produce the effect of lessening the intensity of masking environmental sounds. Similarly, a cold may produce a stiffness in the middle ear mechanisms, which then induces tinnitus through increased internal reflections.

VIRAL INFECTIONS

Behçet's disease is a chronic multisystemic disorder, thought to be virally caused, that mainly affects young adults and is characterised by a relapsing inflammatory process. Tinnitus in Behçet's syndrome is not uncommon. Brama and Fainaru (1980) noted that inner ear involvement is a late complication of the disease,

146

often appearing almost a decade after the initial manifestations. Tinnitus can also be a symptom in herpes zoster (Ramsay Hunt syndrome), which is caused by the same viral infection as chickenpox. The virus settles around sensory nerve cells about to enter the spinal cord and causes painful blisters in the areas of skin served by the affected nerves, commonly the face and ear. The virus can cause deafness.

OTOMASTOIDITIS

The mastoid process is a spongy air-filled bone behind the ear that in mastoiditis becomes inflamed, normally because of the spread of pus or bacteria from an untreated infection of the middle ear. The condition is painful and causes fever and deafness. Goodhill (1981) points out that the damage done can cause various fluids to leak into the middle ear and inner ear, which might cause tinnitus.

FEVER (PYREXIA)

Hazell (1981a) points out that tinnitus can be a symptom in persons who are feverish. Fever is usually a symptom of a bacterial or viral infection.

MENINGITIS

McFadden (1982), summarising others, points out that a general medical examination of the individual with tinnitus should exclude meningitis as a possible cause. Meningitis is a disease caused by inflammation of the meninges (the three membranes that enclose the brain and spinal cord) due to viral infections and other causes.

LABYRINTHITIS

The labyrinth is the structure and mechanism in the inner ear that controls balance. It can succumb to viral and bacterial infections originating elsewhere but passing up the eustachian tube; loss of balance and dizziness, as well as tinnitus, may ensue. In some cases the damage done may cause fluid leaks between areas in the inner ear and the middle ear, with in some instances a resulting tinnitus. Meyerhoff and Shrewsbury (1980) consider that tinnitus in labyrinthitis may also have allergic or spirochaetal origins.

MIGRAINE

Migraines are severe recurrent, often one-sided, headaches sometimes accompanied by visual disturbances as well as an inability to tolerate light — there are many other associated symptoms. Migraines are caused by excessive sensitivity of the blood vessels in the head; initially arteries and capillaries within the skull contract, and then they widen. A whole variety of factors may trigger off an attack. Martin (1982) mentions that tinnitus may be associated with migrainous tendency, and McFadden (1982) places it on his list of things to be taken account of in the medical examination of the tinnitus patient.

HYPERTENSION

Meyerhoff and Shrewsbury (1980) list consistently high blood pressure as a factor that may be associated with tinnitus, and changes in the blood supply in the small vessels serving the inner ear may influence tinnitus. Meyerhoff and Shrewsbury also suggest that tinnitus may be associated with *arteriosclerotic heart disease* — the hardening of the arteries around the heart that is a normal part of the gradual process of ageing. The arterial walls become hardened by the deposition of calcium, and thickened as the result of the long-term effects of raised blood pressure. McFadden (1982) also suggests that a check should be made to see if *vasospastic disease* is present, in which blood vessels undergo spasms — contractions and dilations — as in migraine attacks.

KIDNEY FUNCTION

McFadden (1982) points out that the ear is commonly asserted to be like the kidney in that both structures are concerned with maintaining normal electrolyte concentration gradients. Each electrolyte — be it sodium, potassium, chlorine, calcium, etc. — circulates in the body in the form of electrically charged particles, known as ions, some of which are charged positively (sodium, for example). The health of the body and its processes depends on the balance between the two charges, because they provide the necessary electrical environment for chemical reactions to take place. Sodium and potassium are particularly important because nerve impulses are unable to move along nerve fibres without them. The similarity between the kidney and the ear in this respect causes them to react similarly to certain agents. Thus McFadden (1982) suggests that normal kidney function should be established in sufferers from severe tinnitus.

SERUM LIPIDS

These are fat-like substances, such as cholesterol, in the blood. Hazell (1981a) suggests that hyperlipidaemia, a systemic disease in which there is excess fat in the blood, should be excluded when a patient presents with tinnitus. High blood levels of lipids may be indicative of conditions such as diabetes and liver and thyroid disorders.

AUTOIMMUNE DISORDERS

There are a group of diseases that are thought to be caused to some degree by a malfunction of the immune system, which is part of the natural defence system of the body against foreign organisms. Normally the body's immune system recognises a foreign invader as potentially harmful and produces antibodies to fight it. Problems in the autoimmune system may lead antibodies to attack the body's own tissues. Various disorders may be connected with autoimmune problems: thyroiditis, AIDS, diabetes, rheumatoid arthritis, and perhaps multiple sclerosis. McFadden (1982) suggests that the complete medical examination of the tinnitus sufferer should include a check-up on the immune system.

NERVE COMPRESSION

Mathur (1980) hypothesises that tinnitus, vertigo (dizziness) and nerve deafness might follow from compression by blood vessels of the vestibulocochlear nerve — the eighth cranial nerve, concerned with hearing and balance.

BELL'S PALSY

Bell's palsy has also been considered capable of producing tinnitus (Meyerhoff and Shrewsbury 1980). In this condition, which has as yet no known cause, one of the two facial (seventh cranial) nerves swells up within its canal. The wall of the canal constricts the swollen nerve to cause a paralysis of the muscles on the side of the face supplied by the affected nerves.

OTOSCLEROSIS

Meyerhoff and Shrewsbury (1980) list otosclerosis as one of a variety of conditions that cause or are associated with tinnitus. Otosclerosis usually develops in late adolescence and is hereditary in 50 per cent of cases. It causes a thickening of the tiny bones in the middle ear, which results in their decreasing ability to transmit vibration across from the ear drum to the inner ear and hence results in hearing loss. As well as tinnitus, vertigo may also result from otosclerosis.

JAW JOINT DEFECTS

Martin (1982) suggests that in some instances tinnitus is associated with jaw joint dysfunction. Brookes *et al.* (1980), however, consider that the tinnitus that may appear in Costen's syndrome is coincidental and not directly related to the jaw joint dysfunction that may produce otalgia — a form of ear pain originating in the nerves.

HEAD INJURY

Tinnitus is not an uncommon consequence of severe head injury but a predisposition to hearing loss and tinnitus probably pre-exists when instances of *mild* head injury seem to be associated with tinnitus onset. Goodhill (1981) suggests that head traumas may lead to fluid leakage in the middle and inner ear, and hence to tinnitus.

TUMOURS AND NEUROMAS

A tumour is an abnormal growth of cells in the body. Those developing in or near the ear are in most instances harmless (benign) in that they are not malignant, i.e. they are not showing the uncontrolled growth of cancerous cells. Neuromas are benign tumours that develop in the fibrous sheath covering a nerve. An acoustic neuroma is one that compresses the eighth cranial nerve, which supplies the ears. The main symptom of this is tinnitus with vertigo, unilateral tinnitus being the presenting symptom in 8 to 10 per cent of cases (Hazell 1981a).

DRUGS CAUSING OR EXACERBATING TINNITUS

At the CIBA Symposium on Tinnitus, Tonndorf asked — 'Is there any class of drugs that has *not* generally been reported to produce tinnitus?' (in Evered and Lawrenson 1981, p. 169). Brown *et al.* (1981) list some 50 drugs thought to produce tinnitus that also cause temporary or permanent hearing loss when given in certain dosages. They produce an additional list of some 67 drugs thought to produce tinnitus that do not seem to cause hearing loss. Hazell (1979c) reports that 11 per cent of his subjects with tinnitus had taken drugs at one time or another that could have had a damaging effect on the ear. In this section we shall pay attention to a small selection of drugs, some of which are in relatively common use and some of which have been more recently reported to produce or exacerbate tinnitus.

Antibiotics

These are drugs that fight bacterial infection. Broad-spectrum antibiotics are active against a variety of bacteria while others are active only against specific species or strains. Some kill bacteria while others stop them reproducing. They are not active against viral infections. Several antibiotics have been linked to production of tinnitus in susceptible individuals: kanamycin, vancomycin, neomycin, deoxycyclinex, erythromycin, chloramphenicol and streptomycin.

Pain-killers, fever and inflammation reducers

By far the most commonly used drugs in this class is aspirin, high doses of which will produce tinnitus in almost everyone. There is little evidence that tinnitus might be a consequence of long periods of taking aspirin at normal doses in normal individuals. There may be instances in which taking aspirin actually alleviates tinnitus. Certainly it is thought that a small dose of aspirin would not produce any *permanent* change in tinnitus. However, Daneshmend (1979) states that tinnitus *can* occur as the sole complaint in low doses in susceptible individuals and suggests that because of its ubiquity it seems wise to exclude the drug as a cause of tinnitus. Similarly, Ronis (1984) advocates a six-week salycilate-free diet to see if this might help and usefully lists those foods that *are* salycilate free. The tinnitus induced by aspirin is usually tonal and of high frequency (McFadden 1982). Both brufen and indomethacin may produce tinnitus.

Anti-depressants

We shall be considering the role of anti-depressants in the *treatment* of tinnitus in a later chapter. Because anti-depressants are widely advocated as part of a treatment regime for tinnitus, it is necessary to be aware that in some susceptible individuals they may produce or exacerbate tinnitus even if in others the tinnitus and anti-depressant treatment is coincidental. Phenelzine is a now less-frequently prescribed anti-depressant that is one of the monoamine oxidase inhibitors. These can react adversely and dangerously with cheese and Chianti wine in particular. Glass (1981) reports the case of an individual who had been taking phenelzine for five weeks when he noticed the onset of intermittent tinnitus. The drug was discontinued and the tinnitus stopped within a week. The now more commonly prescribed tricyclic anti-depressants, for example imipramine, amitriptyline, doxepin and protriptyline, have also been implicated in production or exacerbation of tinnitus (Golden, Evans and Nau 1983).

Some 11 per cent of our respondents were currently using pain-relief and anti-inflammatory drugs and some 6 per cent were taking anti-depressant drugs capable of producing or exacerbating tinnitus in susceptible individuals.

'TREATMENTS' CAUSING OR EXACERBATING TINNITUS

Drugs apart, there are other treatments, mostly to rectify hearing loss or correct problems in or in the vicinity of the ear, that can in some instances cause tinnitus or make an existing tinnitus worse. When such treatments are being considered doctors should be frank with patients as to the possible outcome (a) for the main problem and (b) for the tinnitus, so that individuals can make informed choices before undergoing treatment. The first treatment we shall mention, however, has no role in the treatment of hearing problems, but is mostly used to alleviate very severe forms of depression.

Electro-convulsive therapy (ECT)

The evidence about the effects of ECT on tinnitus are anecdotal, but since some Tinnitus Association Newsletter readers have wondered if it can be used as a *treatment* for tinnitus, it is important to point out its possible detrimental effects and state that it has *no* role in the treatment of tinnitus. The reasons for the effects of ECT on depression are not understood, let alone for its possible effects on tinnitus. There is no real proof that tinnitus is worsened by ECT, but this has been reported. Vernon (in Evered and Lawrenson 1982, p. 230) mentions four patients who had been through electric shock treatment and who 'now have about the most intractable tinnitus that we have seen'.

Auditory nerve section

The auditory nerve is the eighth cranial nerve, which relays messages from the inner ear to the brain about sound and balance. In the ear it divides into two parts, one leading to the cochlea and dealing with sound, the other leading to the balance mechanism — the semicircular canals. The operation to cut the nerve of hearing, or one or other of its two ends in the inner ear, is only undertaken when there is more or less *no* useful hearing in the ear under consideration, and it is undertaken to try and relieve intractable balance disorders that make individuals ill with nausea and dizziness. There seems to be little predictability about the outcome of the operation as far as any particular individual is concerned. Barrs and Brackmann (1984) state that of the 110 patients studied,

153

tinnitus was improved in 61 per cent of those who had the balance *and* hearing parts of the nerve both cut, but only 49 per cent of those having the balance part alone cut showed improvement. Sometimes the auditory nerve is damaged, resulting in tinnitus, in a mastoidectomy operation. Here some of the spongy air-filled bone behind the ear has to be removed so that pus can be drained out and infected bone replaced; this usually is advised when infection has been prolonged and antibiotics ineffective. The operation may also result in a conductive hearing loss, which means that potentially masking external noise is lessened and an existing tinnitus may be heard more clearly.

Acoustic neuroma and tumours

Operations to remove acoustic neuromas can themselves affect any associated tinnitus. Hazell (1981a) reports studies showing that about 50 per cent of those undergoing surgery for an acoustic neuroma have some improvement in their tinnitus.

Stapedectomy

With deafness due to otosclerosis it is often considered that removing the third minute bone in the middle ear (the stapes) and replacing it with a tiny plastic piston will help restore some useful hearing (although a hearing aid may also be needed). House and Brackman (1981) note that successful stapedectomies can be anticipated in 90 per cent of cases as far as improved hearing is concerned, but that tinnitus does not always disappear or improve. It may disappear in roughly 40 per cent of cases, decrease in 34 per cent, not change in 20 per cent and be worse in 3 per cent of cases. However, stapedectomy failures can occur — perhaps in one in 20 operations — with consequent deafness, and the tinnitus following a failed stapedectomy is sometimes of the worst kind.

Surgery in or near the ear

Although the evidence is slight and what there is is anecdotal, it is not difficult to imagine that surgery in the vicinity of the ear may effect tinnitus. Noise exposure during ear or head surgery, for example the noise of drilling or even of surgical instruments dropped on the operating table, might be damaging, especially in surgery in which the protection afforded by the middle ear is missing, which would allow the inner ear to be exposed to substantial noise. That some tinnitus (and hearing loss) may be *iatrogenic* — literally 'caused by doctors' — is not surprising, since treatment for one problem cannot exist in complete isolation from the causation of others. However, the possibility that the various treatments for tinnitus may ultimately prove iatrogenic, i.e. may in the long-term make the tinnitus worse, is something that must be faced.

12

Helping Yourself

One piece of advice that can be given to a person who has newly started with tinnitus, which is a variation on the 'learn to live with it' theme, is to 'stick with it', because we *know* that people *can* and *do* come to terms and successfully live with quite severe forms of tinnitus. To some 'new' sufferers this might be hard to believe. Hazell (1979a) points out that what is surprising is not the fact that some people are driven to desperation by their tinnitus but rather how many sufferers *do* manage to adapt and adjust to their tinnitus. He considers that such adaptation takes from six months to a year, and that after that any further adaptation to or ability to cope better with the tinnitus is less likely — though this seems to us to be an over-pessimistic view.

LESSENING WORRIES

In an earlier chapter we remarked that tinnitus tended to be rated louder the longer a person has it, irrespective of his or her actual age, and that tinnitus in older people tended to be rated louder irrespective of the length of time they had had it. We also noted that these differences in loudness (as tapped by our two loudness rating scales) were quite small, so that individuals should not worry about their tinnitus getting worse. If our results had shown on average that, say, in a ten-year period with tinnitus, a loudness rating moved from 'water simmering on a pot' to 'thunder clap overhead', then there would be cause for concern. The fact that tinnitus, when rated, might seem louder the longer the individual has had it, does not mean that it plays an increasingly objectionable role in his or her life, since, on the contrary, over the years for most people, in the

156

majority of circumstances and most of the time, the tinnitus becomes part of the environment — a sort of 'noise wallpaper', the existence of which is taken for granted, and the annoyance from which only dominates from time to time.

We asked our respondents to tell us what worried them about their tinnitus. Although just under three-quarters of our respondents listed at least one worry, one in ten stated that they had no worries, and one in twelve actually volunteered that they had 'learned to live with it' even though the question was asking them to state their *worries*. Another one in twelve considered the tinnitus to be more of an irritation than a worry. When we examined how the proportions of those stating that they had no worries varied according to the length of time they had had tinnitus, we found that significantly fewer of those who had had tinnitus longest reported having worries, i.e. the longer the individual had had the tinnitus the more likely he or she was to report *not* having any worries about it ($\chi^2 = 3.866$, $df = 1$, $P = 0.049$). Similarly, older respondents were significantly more likely than younger ones to report 'no worries' about their tinnitus ($\chi^2 = 4.162$, $df = 1$, $P = 0.0413$).

WHAT DO YOU DO THAT HELPS?

We asked our respondents the question 'Is there anything that you do that you have found helps with your tinnitus?' Fifty-three per cent of our respondents replied 'Yes'. Of these, just over one in four mentioned being absorbed in something, be it a hobby, work, or other activities that demanded attention and with which they could become pre-occupied. Nearly one in four of these respondents also suggested 'keeping busy'. Clearly, then, the predominant action undertaken by our respondents to help with their tinnitus was being active and occupied in something or other that they found absorbing. This, of course, suggests that if concentration is firmly focused on one thing it can't be focused so well on another, i.e. on the tinnitus. Nearly one in ten respondents offering suggestions mentioned that 'conversation' or 'being in company' helped. Again these are activities where usually the individual's awareness is focused on others. Just under one in 14 of the respondents who had found things to do that helped with their tinnitus mentioned getting into the open air and going for walks. This might produce both attentional and masking effects on the tinnitus for some individuals, in that outdoors may be noisier than indoors, and that a brisk walk is an activity that enables one to pay regard to a changing environment. It is possible that such an activity might alleviate tension due to feeling claustrophobic or 'house-bound' in some people.

Being very active may be a double-edged sword, as one letter-writer to the British Tinnitus Association points out:

Living with tinnitus

I should be most interested to learn whether others share my experiences and observations with tinnitus.

Severe tinnitus in one ear together with associated inner ear deafness first arrived with me when I was 18. It lasted some three years and then equally suddenly remitted to an extent that neither the tinnitus nor the deafness bothered me seriously. Twelve years ago, both symptoms recurred in a much more severe form and this has been the situation ever since. For a long while during this period I had a very responsible job with a major multinational [company].

My observations are as follows: although I claim to have severe tinnitus there are occasions when the noise virtually disappears. These occasions occur when I am intensely involved in something demanding, such as chairing a difficult meeting or racing my sailing dinghy, and when, presumably, the adrenalin is flowing. However, as night follows day, the tinnitus returns more severely than ever as one begins to relax. For instance, after an evening meeting, I can go to bed with virtually no tinnitus only to wake an hour or so later with no hope of further sleep without resorting to sedation.

Over the years I have made many attempts to 'snap out of it' and live a life of great activity and courage. And it used to work, as sometimes for weeks at a time I was convinced the tinnitus was all in the mind and it was only a question of adopting a sufficiently positive mental approach. However, the length of time I could sustain such periods became shorter and shorter and now I cannot do it at all. After all these years I seem to have got tense and tired and my tolerance to anxiety has reduced. Even quite ordinary physical activity such as walking and gardening seems to aggravate the tinnitus.

After leaving my demanding job about three years ago I did virtually nothing other than jobs around the house and garden for nine months and at the end of that period both the tinnitus and my sleep difficulties had ceased to be a problem, so much so that I can remember throwing away my BTA Newsletter unopened. But I was bored stiff so I began to take on responsibilities again and before long I was back to square one where I still am.

So my experiences are rather conflicting. On the one hand, intense activity and stimulation banishes tinnitus for a while, but the reaction is severe. On the other hand, a prolonged period of freedom from responsibility and stimulation also had a very beneficial effect upon the tinnitus. I suspect the right answer for many sufferers is to find an activity which is interesting and absorbing, preferably involving contact with other people, but yet not *too* stimulating, responsible or demanding. Unfortunately most people are not in a position to readjust their lives in this way and even if you are lucky enough to be able to do so, it is not easy to find the right thing.

D.E. Watts
Tunbridge Wells

As the reader's letter suggests, few individuals will be completely free to change their life to get the activity balance just right. The reader mentions a 'positive mental approach' and 6.5 per cent of our respondents giving suggestions may have been thinking along these lines when they mentioned 'using willpower to ignore the tinnitus'.[1]

Being active may lead to over-activity, over-tiredness, together with an inability to relax or 'wind down'. It is under such circumstances, particularly at the end of the day, that many individuals rate their tinnitus as being at its loudest. Being able to successfuly relax is something to which we shall return in more detail in a later chapter. Here we will note that of those respondents giving helpful suggestions, 8.9 per cent mentioned keeping calm and relaxed, 3.2 per cent mentioned getting into a quiet environment, and 1.4 per cent mentioned lying down quietly. Obviously, partly a factor in these suggestions is a quiet as opposed to a noisy environment. Although most people probably need a quiet (or at least soothing) environment in which to relax, some find a quiet environment enables them to pay more (unwanted) attention to their tinnitus.

Using sound productively

Whereas some respondents sought out a quiet environment, 3.8 per cent of those giving suggestions did the reverse, they actively avoided quiet environments; 3.4 per cent said they created one or other sort of noise around themselves; while 6.9 per cent said they found listening to music helped; and nearly 12 per cent mentioned listening to the radio, cassettes or watching TV. Obviously these latter activities also involve attentional aspects. Some individuals, of course, find that listening to music exacerbates their tinnitus. Such is the idiosyncratic nature of tinnitus that some individuals find a quiet environment helps while others find it exacerbates the problem. On balance, though, the data from our respondents suggest that those finding relief in quiet environments are in the minority.

Sounds giving relief

We asked our respondents to indicate if one or more of four specified sounds gave relief from the tinnitus. The sounds were: music, running water, traffic noises, and whistling or humming to yourself. Forty-eight per cent of our respondents reported that listening to music gave relief — such an activity obviously involves the masking potential of music as well as attentional factors and may also relate to relaxation — people often play music when they are relaxed or to help them relax. Only 23.7 per cent reported getting relief from running water.

We mentioned in an earlier chapter that many people find that traffic noise, as one form of relatively loud noise, exacerbates tinnitus, but in answer to the current question 36.6 per cent of our respondents reported that traffic noise gave them relief. Traffic noise as a factor in relief is largely sound orientated — attention is not involved except for listening for 'oddities' that might indicate something unusual might be happening, as in an accident. Average street traffic noise is between 80 and 90 dB and probably represents a level of loudness that most individuals would find intolerable in a masking device. Surprisingly, as many as one in ten of our respondents said that humming or whistling to oneself gave relief. Perhaps the effect in this instance is that the action of whistling and/or humming gives the brain something else to listen to that may be more pleasant than the tinnitus and that is inherently controllable.

Our respondents were also asked to list any *other* sounds that helped. Their replies were coded into 19 apparently different sorts of noise, although several could be inferred to have elements in common. Just over 40 per cent of the entire sample of respondents listed one or more 'extra' sounds that gave them relief from the tinnitus, and of these the following seemed most significant. *Conversation* was reported by 18.8 per cent of those listing extra sounds. Conversational speech (about 60 dB) is obviously quieter than a business office (65 dB), say, but quite a lot louder than ambient noise in a living-room (about 40 dB). Conversation requires attention and directed listening and this, as well as the *noise* of conversation, must play a part in the relief it brings. Over 4 per cent mentioned the sort of level of noise common at parties or in a crowd of people. The next most common noise, mentioned by 18 per cent was *loud* noise, with noise from machinery often given as an elaboration, while 10.1 per cent said that noises louder than the tinnitus gave relief. Although there is no exact one-to-one relationship between tinnitus loudness and the loudness of a sound required to mask it, it appears that many respondents are aware of masking effects from loud or relatively loud noises. Of those reporting additional sounds, some 14 per cent said that any sound gave them relief, while nearly 9 per cent mentioned 'everyday sounds'. These probably represent the sort of ambient sound levels found in a living room (40 dB) or maybe even those found in a library (37 dB). Also mentioned were: water gushing (2.7 per cent); sea or seashore sounds (3 per cent); and wind (2.7 per cent). Nearly 5 per cent of those mentioning extra sounds that brought relief reported that *deliberate* listening helped, and bracketed with these are the 15.1 per cent who mentioned listening to records, cassettes and the radio, and watching TV. Over 4 per cent mentioned that listening to tapes or records or the radio *through headphones* was particularly effective.

One might expect those who rate their tinnitus as quiet would find that, other things being equal, there are a wider variety of sounds that bring relief than there are for those who rate their tinnitus as loud. This seemed to be the case among our respondents. Of those reporting that loud sounds gave relief, 69 per cent had louder forms of tinnitus (as rated on the adjectival scale as at normal conversation levels or above), whereas 31 per cent had quieter forms of tinnitus; but of those who reported that conversation gave relief, 65 per cent had quieter forms of tinnitus and 35 per cent had louder forms. Relief for louder forms of tinnitus appeared to come from loud noises, water rushing, sea or seashore sounds, and using headphones. One in ten of all our respondents, however, stated that *no* sounds gave them relief.

LIFE-STYLE MANAGEMENT

Some things cannot be changed. If tinnitus is at its worst in the early evening or first thing in the morning, early evenings and breakfast-time cannot be banished as such! But the individual can exert a degree of control over many of the factors that *do* appear to influence tinnitus for the worse. The two most important factors to consider are stress and tiredness, but before considering these we will return to the role that food, drink, drugs and smoking may play, and to tinnitus-lessening activities.

Food, drink and smoking

Giving up smoking is good for you — all smokers know that already. It also gives you extra cash in your pocket, and it *might,* in the long run, help with the tinnitus if only because being healthy and fit helps one cope better with stress. Most smokers are looking for an extra reason to motivate them to start a non-smoking regime — tinnitus sufferers *have* it. It may appear to worsen the tinnitus in the short-term, as nicotine withdrawal symptoms appear and the smoker feels more irritable and 'on-edge' as the craving increases. But in the long-term the now non-smoker is going to feel healthier and wealthier — and his or her tinnitus *may* be less aggravated. Smoking 'to soothe one's nerves' because the tinnitus is bad, might, through conditioning and association, lead to the tinnitus appearing louder on many, if not most, occasions on which the smoker chooses to smoke.

Giving up smoking may not be fun while you are doing it, but altering one's *dietary* routine can be both fun and interesting. One no longer has to scour the back streets of big cities to find food (admittedly still mainly vegetarian) to which *additives* haven't been added. And there are any number of 'whole or health food' recipe books available full of tasty and tempting recipes — and the very activity of preparing and cooking them may help too. Changing diet in this way may not help many people with tinnitus, but it can't do them any harm and it could be good for them. More specifically individuals might take a concerned interest in the effects on their tinnitus of what they eat and drink, and cut out caffeine, quinine and animal fats for a while to see if that helps. In a similar vein it might prove useful to avoid aspirin-based painkillers and use paracetamol instead, as well as being more conscious of the effects that other drugs might be having on the tinnitus. If the tinnitus sufferer thinks there is a connection between a drug he or she is taking and the tinnitus, it should be mentioned to the family doctor, since there may well be alternative drugs to try.

Helpful activities

It makes sense for individuals with tinnitus to actively plan to do things that give them pleasure, that they enjoy and can be absorbed in, and that they feel help alleviate the tinnitus. If you know a vigorous walk by the sea was enjoyable and helpful last time, don't let lethargy set in and the last walk become a fond memory — plan to do it again, soon. Try where possible to avoid those activities that you know are likely to exacerbate the tinnitus. If it helps, walk into town or to the nearest shops wearing ear-plugs to cut out traffic noise; if noise seems to help, think of treating yourself to a portable personal cassette player that you can use in 'too quiet' surroundings. Be prepared to experiment to see if doing certain things helps, without putting so much faith in the activity that disappointment follows if it *doesn't* help. For example, if the act of lying horizontal seems to worsen the tinnitus, see if you can get to sleep in a more upright position by using a few pillows; if noise helps, try a bedside radio that you can tune to a favourite 'noise' — a radio with a head-phone socket and a clock setting that will switch the radio off automatically after an hour or so; or get a small loudspeaker wired into a pillow — you might be able to wire one up for yourself, or get a kind relative to buy you one of the commercially available pillows (some are 'stereo') as a present.

Take more of an *active* interest in helping yourself, without becoming *over*-preoccupied with the tinnitus and with finding ways to relieve it. Above all try to find activities or hobbies that to you are *intrinsically* absorbing, so that you avoid becoming *self*-absorbed. Easier said than done, of course, but it is the first step that is usually the hardest. If you 'couldn't be bothered' to find out what was going on at night school last winter, make the effort to do so this winter. Maybe think of giving those yoga classes a try. The medical adviser to the BTA considers yoga to be one of the best and most effective therapies against the stress and anxiety that everyone experiences in everyday life, and reducing stress certainly does help people to cope with tinnitus. Remember that it is impossible to be active *all* the time, that rest and relaxation *are* needed, but that they too may require effort, ironic as this may seem. We shall discuss this further when considering non-medical 'treatments' for tinnitus.

Tiredness and stress

Tiredness and stress are linked not only in that they both seem to exacerbate tinnitus, but often stress may lead to tiredness, and *vice versa*. If stress involves muscular tension, then body energy is being put at the disposal of the musculature to maintain this tension, and this may not just help deplete energy faster, it can also lead to the muscles themselves literally feeling tired because they have been 'working' at being tense all day. Tiredness often leads to conflicts of interest — you, or someone else, would like to do something, but you just feel 'too tired'; and tiredness and irritability often go hand in hand. The individual with tinnitus might find it useful to consciously examine what stressful elements or tiredness-producing factors there are in his or her life that could be alleviated by one or other reasonable strategy. This necessitates taking time out to 'take stock' rather than just letting routines go on in the same old way.

Not all stress *can* be avoided, nor is it desirable that it should be; if all stress was avoided we would find ourselves wrapped up in metaphorical cotton wool, and many of our pleasures would be denied us too. Some new and challenging situations *are* stressful but we are often pleased to have risen to them when they are over. Nor can tiredness be avoided, but *over*-tiredness may be avoidable in many circumstances. It is normal to have a certain degree of tiredness at the end of a working day, and many pleasurable physical activities lead to a *relaxed* form of tiredness that is conducive to sleep. The problem arises when the individual feels *too* tired to get to sleep. This often means getting to sleep *later* but still having to get up at the same time in the morning. Often people who are 'too tired' to get to sleep at 11 p.m. were probably quite capable of going to sleep at 9 p.m. A change in routine to going to bed early for a few days when one *does* feel ready to sleep might be worth trying.

Many individuals with tinnitus (and many without tinnitus, of course) have marked degrees of tension and anxiety that lead them to turn to others for help. Even individuals with mild forms of tinnitus may first think of 'going to the family doctor for some tablets' without even considering that the stress they feel might be a function of their life-style and that *that* might be amenable to positive change. Family doctors themselves are becoming more reluctant to issue tranquillisers as a 'remedy' for stress, since such drugs only treat the symptoms and not the underlying *cause* of the stress. They may be a useful prop to use while finding out what the underlying causes of the stress are, and while attempting to remove such causes where this is possible, but such drugs cannot be a long-term solution.

LOCAL TINNITUS SELF-HELP GROUPS

One positive step towards learning about tinnitus and by learning about it towards coping with it is to join a National Tinnitus Association. This brings the benefits of up-to-date articles on what's new in the world of tinnitus research, and readers' letters illustrating how people have managed to cope with tinnitus together with other problems — as well as their suggestions for what helps. Another positive step for many individuals might be joining a local self-help group, where this is feasible. The simple act of sharing experiences with others in a similar predicament can help — a trouble shared *can* be a trouble halved. Perhaps inevitably the running of such groups will devolve on to three or four individuals who have the necessary time and energy and enthusiasm. But 'ordinary' members each have their own talents that they can put to use. There are those who are good at fund-raising — who don't mind approaching the managing directors of firms for contributions; there are those who like organising jumble sales, coffee mornings or afternoon teas; those who will organise and collect for raffles; those who can organise a dance or disco; those who are willing to approach local TV, radio and newspapers for publicity. Many members may not want to be involved in such activities, which are largely directed at local group funding and funding further research, but they may be willing to put their experiences on paper for the benefit of others in a *local* tinnitus newsletter.

We have mentioned earlier that membership of a local self-help group may not be suitable for some people, simply because the attention given to tinnitus at group meetings may appear to make their own tinnitus temporarily worse. However, membership of a local group inevitably means that individuals meet others whose tinnitus is worse than their own, whose circumstances are more stressful, but who nevertheless are managing to cope. It encourages the normal desire to be helpful to others in distress, and can help people become outward-looking rather than introspective in consideration of themselves. Self-help groups will not help *all* tinnitus sufferers, but they represent another resource of which the tinnitus sufferer should be aware.[2]

NOTES

1. 'Thinking positively' may work for some individuals and another reader suggests two books that have helped him in this respect: Patience Strong's *Life is for Living*, published in London by Frederick Muller in 1971; and Dale Carnegie's *How to Stop Worrying and Start Living*, published in Kingswood, Surrey, by The World's Work, in 1948. Strong's book has religious overtones, whereas Carnegie's now seems a little dated. Neither book will be everyone's cup of tea, but some people may well find these books useful in helping them to stop worrying and to 'think positively'.

2. Setting up a local tinnitus self-help group may seem a daunting task, but a short article in the local press or interview on the local radio, giving details of the date, time and place of a first 'exploratory' meeting, is likely to result in perhaps 50 or 60 individuals turning up from a local area of 100 to 200,000 people. It might be useful at such a first meeting to have a visiting speaker — perhaps someone from the local medical community, or perhaps someone who has some specialist knowledge or interest in tinnitus, or even a local ENT consultant who is willing to explain the complexity of the hearing mechanism in layman's terms and hint at the inherent complexities of the possible tinnitus-producing mechanisms. Perhaps having the secretary or chairman of another established local group come to speak would be helpful. Certainly at such a first meeting the names and addresses of those present should be collected so that any further communications about the group can be sent direct to them, and hopefully a chairman, secretary, treasurer, publicity officer, and fund-raising co-ordinator might be appointed for a provisional term of one year. Better still, a small donation to cover the cost of the initial publicity and the hire of the room, plus that anticipated for the next meeting, should be collected by the treasurer. And time should be allowed for people to meet each other and chat together over tea or coffee. In this manner groups will develop a pattern and style of meetings that seems most appropriate for their own members and their circumstances.

Publicity about the existence of the group and its meetings will be important. It may be useful to get posters put up in appropriate 'public' places — libraries, doctors' surgeries and health clinics, ENT departments and hospital notice boards, as well as news items in the local press and on local radio about forthcoming meetings. As many of these activities as possible should be delegated to group members, so that each has a sense of contributing something.

13

Drug Treatment

RESEARCH PROBLEMS

Many of the drug treatments to be considered in this chapter have 'success rates' for reducing tinnitus, either directly or in terms of its noticeability, that are far from clear cut. Some individuals remain fairly sceptical about drug 'successes', largely because of the methodological difficulties inherent in running drug trials in tinnitus research that are not immune to criticism. As we shall see, even in apparently successful drug trials, we can still only *hypothesise* how the drugs are having their effects. It would be foolish to pretend that there is some wonder-drug or other 'just around the corner', but no doubt our understanding of the many and varied causes of tinnitus will be slowly built up, and with that knowledge will come improvements in the drug treatments that can be offered.

Cathcart (1982), after conducting a drug study on tinnitus, raises the significant question as to whether better results can be obtained from firm reassurance (after initial medical investigations have revealed no problems) than from the use of any drugs yet available that can be given by mouth. This really raises the question of what attempts should be made to give relief *before* drugs are resorted to. Wood *et al.* (1983) think it possible that some individuals might be receptive to *any* specialised treatment techniques for tinnitus. Before considering those drugs that *do* seem effective (given various major constraints) with many people, we should point out a few of the problems inherent in conducting drug trials.

Placebo effects

Marks, Onisiphorou and Trounce (1981) point out the need to take the general variability of loudness estimates into account when conducting drug trials on tinnitus. Because tinnitus is *subjective* (in the vast majority of cases), there is a specific possibility (if not likelihood) of *placebo* effects. A placebo is a 'remedy' without any direct action on a disease or symptom. Many studies have shown that some three-quarters of all patients feel better after taking placebos providing that they *believe* the placebos are active medicines, and in some cases they may actually *be* better. In drug trials with tinnitus, placebos will be given to ensure that the effects of a drug under trial are not simply due to the effects that taking anything (in the belief it is active medicine) would have.

Cathcart (1982), in one drug trial, reports two patients who continued to get apparent relief from a placebo over a period of three months, with no side effects, and suggests that, since tinnitus engenders much anxiety in some individuals, the very act of doing *something* may help. In a similar vein, McFadden (1982) points out that when some people have been through months or years of frustration trying to get relief from their tinnitus, it may be that anyone doing anything in an attempt to help them might be met with reports of success. This element must be built into drug trial methodology, and Majumdar *et al.* (1983), in their drug trial, discounted as 'improvements in tinnitus' any report on a 100 per cent scale for measuring tinnitus level of improvement that said improvement was less than 20 per cent, since 13 of 15 patients reported this degree of improvement after injections with a placebo — salt solution — and three of 20 patients reported even higher levels of improvement after injections of salt solution.

Others have expressed surprise at how *little* such placebo effects are, given that tinnitus *is* such a subjective phenomenon. McCormick and Thomas (1981), for example, drew attention to the *lack* of placebo response that they observed, which suggests, they consider, that tinnitus is not really subjective at all, but is simply relegated under that (somewhat dismissive) terminology, simply because of our inability to demonstrate that it is *objective*. Tinnitus, as almost all 'sufferers' will attest, is a very 'hard' symptom; it is only *too* real and concrete to those who experience it, and to that extent it may be resistant to suggestion and to placebo tablets in most people. Goodey (1981) points out that in his experience people with tinnitus do not in general respond to placebos, and, though he used several different sorts, including salt solution, he reports finding none that have suppressed the tinnitus. One subject of Goodey's reported that salt solution (saline) *reduced* the tinnitus, nevertheless this subject appeared to have the same level of tinnitus when this was measured audiometrically — i.e. as objectively as possible.

Complications in the methodology of drug trials apart, there are also ethical issues. Many of the drugs so far used have known and sometimes severe side-effects, and are primarily intended for treatment of complaints other than tinnitus. Kay (1981), for example, reports of one trial (with volunteers) in which a subject fainted due to sudden loss of blood pressure (a vasovagal attack) on consuming the trial drug, which would normally have been given to people with disorders of heart rhythm. Kay points out that this event exposes the dangers of using a cardiovascular drug for a non-cardiovascular condition. On ethical grounds it was decided that the drug trial would stop, but similar trials with the same drug would necessitate screening out individuals with untoward cardiovascular histories.

LIGNOCAINE (LIDOCAINE) AND ITS DERIVATIVES

Lignocaine or lidocaine (Xylocaine and others) is a local anaesthetic that has also been used to treat disorders of heart rhythm. It may be rubbed on to the skin, which it penetrates well to reach local nerve endings and block pain, or it can be injected to produce a regional nerve block — i.e. to remove pain in a defined area, as when used by dentists. Lignocaine may also be injected into a vein to produce general anaesthesia and it has to be injected to produce an effect on tinnitus. Jackson remarks that the effect of lignocaine, when it works, can be so dramatic in reducing the tinnitus that patients sometimes dissolve into tears of joy at the relief from the noise for the first time in years! (Evered and Lawrenson 1981, pp. 276–7) Lignocaine may not work with individuals who have had tinnitus for more than five years or so and it appears to be least effective in individuals who have normal hearing (Martin and Colman 1980; Goodey 1981) and perhaps more effective on individuals with tinnitus in both ears (McFadden 1982). Majumdar et al. (1983) report significant temporary improvement in the tinnitus in 13 of 20 patients, which confirms the suggestion of others that lignocaine may have an effect on at least 60 per cent of tinnitus sufferers (Hazell 1980b). In perhaps 30 per cent of cases it may abolish the tinnitus completely, and although its effects are usually short, a matter of 20 minutes or so, it can bring relief for days in some individuals (Hazell 1980a). Majumdar et al. (1983) suggest that the effects of lignocaine may be more pronounced in patients with high-pitched tinnitus.

Martin (1980) reported from his drug trial that not only did ligno-caine reduce tinnitus, but it also seemed to lower the tinnitus pitch while active. In this study Martin used both patients' reports of changes in tinnitus and also audiometric equipment to enable him to obtain more objective measures of loudness estimation, the latter also showing a reduced intensity of tinnitus following lignocaine injection. Martin suggests that his findings indicate that psychological factors play a less significant role in tinnitus than was previously thought, or that lignocaine is more effective on changes at the *ends* of the sensorineural hearing system, than on those that may have taken place more centrally in the brain.

Elsewhere Martin (1982) refers to studies showing that in guinea-pigs injection of lignocaine reduced some measurable forms of electrical activity in the ear (the cochlear microphonic and action potential), and Majumdar *et al.* (1983) report reduction of the action potential in human subjects. They argue that tinnitus is reduced as a direct result of altered conductivity in the nerve transmission of auditory signals. They go on to suggest that when lignocaine *is* effective, the place where tinnitus is generated is peripheral, arising in the cochlea itself or possibly in the nerve from the cochlea and that central causation is implicated where lignocaine is ineffective. Martin (1982) also considers that there must be a central brain process component in some cases of persistent tinnitus, since cases are known in which the tinnitus continues even when the primary condition causing the tinnitus has been reversed.

Lignocaine may, then, act either peripherally or centrally, probably by prolonging the time between which nerves can send out impulses. This means that nerves have a reduced ability to fire rapidly or as near as possible to continuously when influenced by lignocaine. Lignocaine is thought, in some forms of tinnitus, to be directly effective on hair cell function in the cochlea, having the effect of making the cell membrane — the outer surface of the cell — more stable; this may make such cells less 'leaky' in ion flow.

Lignocaine can only be administered by *injection* to have any effect on tinnitus, and though its effects have been well demonstrated on individuals with severe and otherwise intractable forms of tinnitus, because its effects are so short-lasting it is thought by some to be impractical to use it as a drug in any continuous forms of treat-ment for tinnitus.

However, Shea (1984) reports giving 500 mg of Xylocaine (lignocaine) per day intravenously for four or five days, repeated weekly in some individuals, together with the long-acting major tranquilliser perphenazine and the mood elevator amitryptiline (contained in the drug Etrafon), as a successful regime for certain individuals. But because many individuals may find such regimes unpalatable, attention has been given to *oral* forms of lignocaine, i.e. those that can be taken by mouth rather than only by injection. One such drug is procaine amide (Pronestyl), which is used in disorders of heart rhythm. Martin (1982) reports that it has some effect on tinnitus in a handful of cases. Tocainide hydrochloride (Tonocard) is a local anaesthetic like lignocaine but it can be given orally. It is not as effective in reducing tinnitus as lignocaine (McFadden 1982), but even if ineffective itself on some individuals it may sometimes enhance the therapeutic effectiveness of masking (Hazell 1981d). Shea, Emmet, Orchick, Mays and Webb (1981) suggest that some individuals who respond well to lignocaine may be maintained on tocainide supplemented with relatively small doses of perphenazine.

Shea (1984) reports using dosages of tocainide — 400 mg taken up to four times a day — without adverse effects, but Hulshof and Vermey (1984) suggest no more than 900 mg of tocainide should be taken per day in total. Cathcart (1982), however, in a drug trial of tocainide, concluded that it did not offer much hope in the relief of tinnitus aurium. Many patients have been reported to have severe side effects from tocainide, and there is little evidence that it would be of help to the majority of sufferers. Mexiletine is another drug similar to lignocaine that can be taken by mouth and is used to treat disorders of heart rhythm. McCormick and Thomas (1981) report it to be ineffective for the relief of tinnitus as a result of a drug trial they conducted. A similar finding was reported by Kay (1981).

Hazell (1984a) reports that lignocaine analogues that can be taken by mouth are still being prescribed in the USA in quite large amounts, even though the results of controlled trials continue to be disappointing. No doubt this partly reflects desperation, on the part of both the doctor and the patient — a feeling that anything is worth a try.

CARBAMAZEPINE AND OTHER ANTICONVULSANT DRUGS

Carbamazepine (Tegretol) is an anticonvulsant drug used mainly in the treatment of epilepsy and sometimes in the treatment of facial or central pain (trigeminal neuralgia). Its recognised adverse effects are dryness of the mouth, nausea, diarrhoea, dizziness and double vision. Sometimes it produces skin rashes, blood disorders and jaundice, which may be indicative of liver damage. When taken by mouth for tinnitus, such large doses have been necessary for unpleasant side effects to be fairly common (Hazell 1980a). It works best on individuals who have marked relief of tinnitus from lignocaine, and in one trial, of those patients who got complete relief from lignocaine, over two-thirds obtained more than 60 per cent relief (total relief being 100 per cent) with carbamazepine. Some individuals, however, may respond to carbamazepine even though lignocaine has no effect on their tinnitus (Martin 1982) although the evidence is conflicting.

In requisite doses carbamazepine may depress the white cell count in the blood (those cells that attack foreign organisms), and can produce liver and kidney damage. For these reasons patients taking carbamazepine have to have their blood and liver function regularly tested, although nausea and vomiting seem to be the main side effects. If carbamazepine seems ineffective, its effect may be enhanced in some individuals by the use of a tricyclic antidepressant; the two drugs sometimes seem to have a synergistic effect on tinnitus — working well together but not necessarily so well separately. Martin (1982) reports finding carbamazepine to be only of occasional benefit, and Marks et al. (1981) found no effect from a single oral dose, although they suggest repeat doses might have been effective. Similarly Donaldson (1981), following a low-dose drug trial, suggests that the initial excitement over the effects of carbamazepine may have been premature; one in five of his patients, even on low doses, could not tolerate the drug because of its adverse side effects.

Melding and Goodey (1979) suggest that tinnitus can be thought of as analogous to epilepsy. In epilepsy, which is an abnormality of brain function, electrical discharges of unusually high voltage occur periodically in the brain tissue. Most epilepsy, like most tinnitus, is idiopathic, in that the actual cause is unknown. Tinnitus might in some cases be a form of sensory epilepsy and Melding and Goodey speculate that it is a manifestation of spontaneous over-activity in certain central pathways of the brain, rather than at the periphery in the ear. Shea and Harell (1978) report one case in which a small dose of carbamazepine gave complete relief to an objective form of tinnitus — palatal myoclonus, but Toland, Porbubsky, Coker and Adams (1984) consider that there is no 'drug of choice' in the treatment of the condition.

Shea and Emmet (1981), noting the serious side effects from carbamazepine, decided to try another short-acting oral anticonvulsant drug used to treat major epileptic attacks — primidone (Mysoline). Their results with primidone were reported to be much the same as with carbamazepine, except for less-serious side effects, and for that reason it was generally considered more satisfactory. The usual dose was 250 mg given daily for the first week, 250 mg twice-daily for the second week, 250 mg three times daily the third week, and finally 250 mg four times daily in the fourth week, until a good response in tinnitus reduction had been obtained. Blood disorders and liver damage following from primidone are very rare, so blood counts and liver function tests do not need to be monitored with primidone as they do with carbamazepine. Martin (1982) mentioned another anticonvulsant drug, phenytoin (Epanutin, Dilantin), used for epilepsy treatment, which has been tried for its effect on tinnitus; it is considered less effective than carbamazepine but it has fewer side effects. Sodium valproate (Epilim, Depakene) is another anticonvulsant drug used in epilepsy treatment, and Martin (1982) reported that in individuals who have a good response to lignocaine it may have an effect on tinnitus similar to that of carbamazepine, although its side effects — drowsiness and occasional indigestion — are fewer.

OTHER DRUGS CONSIDERED IN THE TREATMENT OF TINNITUS

Sodium amylobarbitone (sodium Amytal) and amylobarbitone (Amytal) are barbiturates used in small doses to calm people down, i.e. as a sedative, and in large doses to help them get to sleep, i.e. as a hypnotic; they are also used in the treatment of epilepsy. Donaldson (1978) reported that eleven of twelve patients with severe tinnitus benefited from a sodium amylobarbitone regime, and that for two of these individuals the tinnitus was actually abolished. The drug can, however, be addictive and cause liver damage in some instances. Marks et al. (1981), using single oral doses of amylobarbitone, were unable to demonstrate any effect on tinnitus, although they admit that repeated doses might have proven effective.

Tricyclic antidepressants (e.g. amitriptyline hydrochloride; Lentizol, Triptizol, Amavil, Amitid) may adversely effect the tinnitus in certain individuals, but it is possible that they may have a direct positive effect on the tinnitus in others. Goodey (1981) suggests they have an anticonvulsant as well as an antidepressant action, and reports that some of his patients have found the drugs not only helping them to be more able to tolerate the tinnitus, but also finding that it actually reduces it. In these cases the *residual* tinnitus could be suppressed by intravenous lignocaine, and Goodey suggests this is indicative of the anticonvulsant action of the tricyclic drugs and may prove to be of therapeutic significance.

Glutamic acid (Glutacid, Acidulin) and glutamic acid diethylester, in certain injected dosage sequences have been reported by Ehrenberger and Brix (1983) to have an objectively demonstrable effect on tinnitus. Glutamic acid is an amino acid that can be taken by mouth and is used to reduce minor epileptic attacks as well as to increase mental and physical awareness in mentally handicapped individuals. Glutamic acid is thought to be one of the prime agents involved in nerve signal transmission in the inner ears of mammals, and the diethylester can inhibit its operation. Ehrenberg reports that long-term suppression of certain forms of tinnitus was observed depending on the sequence in which the two substances were injected and on the speed and quantity injected. He suggests that results indicate that tinnitus generated *peripherally* can be influenced by substances altering the chemical transmission capacities of cochlear structures. As with any treatment involving frequent injections, the drugs in their present form are unlikely to prove of substantial help to many tinnitus sufferers. Nicotinic acid (Niacin, Nico-400), like alcohol, is a vasodilator, that is a drug used to improve blood circulation by widening the arterial blood vessels. If individuals find that alcohol helps reduce the noticeability of their tinnitus (directly, rather than because of its sedative effects), it is possible they may obtain the same effect from nicotinic acid. Sometimes the dose has to be raised to a level that causes the face to begin to flush, as the blood supply to it (and to the ears) is increased, but on the whole the drug is relatively harmless, although there are some known side effects, such as nausea and vomiting.

Naftidrofuryl oxilate (Praxilene) is another vasodilator used for the treatment of blood circulation disorders, particularly those affecting the extremities and the circulation system in the head, but it has to be given intravenously to effect tinnitus. Hazell (1980a) reports that although some spectacular results were achieved earlier on, with one patient being without tinnitus for a matter of some months, the drug awaits further wide-scale testing. Because of the need to inject it and its side effects, the drug in its present form is unlikely to be of use to all but a handful of tinnitus sufferers.

DRUGS GIVEN TO HELP INDIVIDUALS COPE WITH TINNITUS

Any individual with severe tinnitus of sudden onset may well feel depressed, anxious, and be suffering from loss of sleep; accordingly a doctor might prescribe tranquillisers, antidepressants, or sleeping tablets, depending on which symptom seems most in need of alleviation. Although anxiety may be the dominant presenting problem apart from the tinnitus, in most cases depression is likely to be an underlying component in many individuals. The medical adviser to the British Tinnitus Association suggests that on the whole it is not advisable that people with tinnitus take tranquillisers if it can at all be avoided, and Kay (1981) found that diazepam, the most commonly prescribed tranquilliser (Valium, Atensine), had no direct effect on the tinnitus in a drug trial he undertook. However, Lechtenberg and Shulman (1984) report that 69 per cent of a small sample of tinnitus sufferers given clonezapam (Rivotril — a minor tranquilliser) in 0.5 mg doses three times a day, considered that the drug had lessened the tinnitus; four individuals reported complete or nearly complete resolution of the tinnitus. The drug in this dosage caused little drowsiness as a side effect. They suggest that this effect is due to the anticonvulsant properties of clonezapam.

Nearly one in five of the respondents in our survey were receiving tranquillisers and respondents with louder forms of tinnitus were significantly more likely to be on such regimes than those with quieter forms of tinnitus ($\chi^2 = 13.78$, $df = 1$, $P < 0.0002$). Similarly, significantly more of those using tranquillisers than one would expect on a chance basis reported difficulties getting to sleep because of the tinnitus ($\chi^2 = 30.24$, $df = 1$, $P < 0.0001$), and difficulty getting to sleep every night of the week ($\chi^2 = 4.096$, $df = 1$, $P < 0.043$), as well as that the tinnitus woke them up ($\chi^2 = 26.189$, $df = 1$, $P < 0.0001$). They were also more likely to report getting headaches often ($\chi^2 = 4.197$, $df = 1$, $P < 0.0405$), as well as getting a headache every day of the week ($\chi^2 = 6.477$, $df = 1$, $P < 0.0109$).

It is hard to tell from these data just how well the tranquillisers helped individuals cope, but those currently receiving tranquillisers still seemed to have a variety of associated problem symptoms, so, if the drugs were helping, these symptoms must have been even more pronounced before the drug treatment commenced. It is significant, though, that louder forms of tinnitus (as self-rated) are associated, as one might intuitively have expected, with a higher incidence of tranquilliser use. Those with the worst forms of tinnitus, as self-perceived, might well be expected to be the most anxious. Yet Hallam *et al.* (1984) suggest that tranquillising and sedating drugs might have paradoxical short- and long-term effects, i.e. help in the short-term, but exacerbate the problem in the long-term. For this reason it might be sensible for those receiving tranquillising drugs to consider with their doctor whether other medication, perhaps anti-depressants, might be more suitable.

We have noted earlier that tricyclic antidepressants not only have been demonstrated to help individuals cope with tinnitus but that they may also, in some instances, help directly alleviate the tinnitus (though making it worse in some others). Among our survey respondents, louder forms of tinnitus were associated with a higher incidence of taking antidepressants, but the significance of this was less marked than for those receiving tranquillisers ($\chi^2 = 3.92$, $df = 1, P < 0.0476$). Apart from also having difficulties getting to sleep (but again to a lesser extent than for those receiving tranquillisers ($\chi^2 = 5.72$, $df = 1$, $P < 0.0167$)), those on antidepressants showed no significant association with the other symptoms significantly associated with those using tranquillisers. Although there is no evidence that sleeping tablets make tinnitus worse, the 'symptom-picture' of our respondents taking sleeping tablets was much more akin to that of those individuals taking tranquillisers than it was to those taking antidepressants. Although it might be the case that respondents with much more severe and intractable forms of tinnitus are given tranquillisers and sleeping tablets rather than antidepressants, it could be the case that antidepressants have the most influential effect in reduction of symptoms.

We are all only too familiar with being 'given a pill' for our ailments and thus many tinnitus sufferers are surprised that there isn't 'a pill' for tinnitus. The complexities of the condition suggest that, in a piecemeal fashion, some drugs *will* be found that can usefully be taken for some forms of tinnitus. However, the day of *the* pill for tinnitus is far off.

14

Psychologically Related Treatments and Therapies

THE 'FIGHT OR FLIGHT' RESPONSE

Physiologically our nervous system evolved so that in moments of perceived danger the body could be quickly mobilised to run away — 'flight' — or to attack — 'fight'. The part of the nervous system under conscious voluntary control makes the decision as to whether the situation is dangerous and whether fight or flight is in order, but it is the unconscious involuntarily controlled *autonomic* nervous system that comes into play to gear up the body for either form of action. The sympathetic nervous system is that part of the autonomic nervous system that sets the body up for action, and the parasympathetic system comes into play after the danger has passed, to bring the body back from its highly aroused state to its normal state.

The main dangers mankind faced as he evolved were attacks from other humans and from animals, as well as those presented by a relatively harsh and uncontrolled physical environment. The main requirements of the body under such circumstances were speed and physical strength, which in essence means maximising energy output to the muscles. For this the muscles need large supplies of food, glucose, and oxygen to help convert the food to energy. To this end the sympathetic nervous system increased the heart rate, so more blood per second is being supplied, it widens the tiny tubes in the lungs (the bronchi) where oxygen enters the bloodstream, so that more oxygen enters, and it widens the arteries carrying the blood to the muscles, so more blood can reach them.

The 'fight or flight' response helped the bodies of primitive man take *physical* action to avoid external *physical* dangers, and so it is the case with modern man under relatively unusual circumstances — running away from a mugger or attacking back, avoiding being knocked down by a car, or helping someone else seen to be in physical danger. But many, if not the majority, of 'dangers' faced by modern man are *psychological* stressors, for which a *physical* bodily response is largely inappropriate.

The consequences of such stress reactions over time may show up more physiologically than psychologically. Psychologically one might *habituate* or get used to stress to such an extent that it is almost taken for granted as one forgets what *relaxation* feels like. The body though, especially the heart, is likely to suffer from being continually pushed to work harder than necessary. If blood pressure is continuously raised, the blood vessels themselves can clog up and harden (atherosclerosis), which lessens blood supply to the tissues, so a vicious circle is set up and the heart has to work even harder to get oxygen supplies through; strokes and heart attacks are potential end products. Because stress reactions also affect the digestive system, another consequence can be ulcerated stomachs and constipation. Over-stressed people may have difficulty getting to sleep, through 'turning things over and over' in their minds, and the sleep they *do* have may be restless, leaving them still tired the next morning. Because a continued stress reaction also reduces the body's internal defence mechanisms against internal attack by foreign invaders such as bacteria and viruses, the over-stressed individual is likely to be more prone to illness, colds and 'flu for example, than is the average person.

Two treatment techniques focus on stress reduction, but in one, biofeedback, the emphasis may be on one of a variety of physiological changes involved in the 'fight or flight' reaction, whereas in progressive relaxation techniques the focus is mainly on tension in the musculature.

BIOFEEDBACK

Biofeedback, as the word implies, involves feeding back to the individual some information about his or her biological (physiological) state. Sometimes it relies on quite complicated electronic monitoring equipment that would normally have to be used in a hospital or clinic setting, but other biofeedback devices are compact enough to be held completely in the hand. The most complicated form of feedback uses information about the electrical activity of the brain.

Slightly less complicated feedback systems have been constructed to give information about electrical activity in particular muscle groups — for example in the muscles of the forehead that make us frown. Less complicated still is skin temperature feedback. The voltage or electrical resistance of certain devices (thermocouples and thermistors) various systematically with changes in temperature, so these can be attached, to a finger say, and information about the skin temperature of the finger can be fed back. Other fairly simple devices, some of which may be completely hand-held, measure the resistance of the skin to electrical current.

In addition, in clinic settings with more complex equipment it is possible to feedback to an individual information about his or her heart rate, blood flow and blood pressure. All of these sources of information have a bearing on the state of the body *vis à vis* 'flight or fight'. When the sympathetic nervous system is functioning, heart rate, blood flow and blood pressure may all increase, brain rhythms will change, muscle activity will increase, skin temperature will drop (as the blood is diverted from the skin to the muscles), and skin resistance to electricity will reduce as sweating starts.

Biofeedback for tinnitus sufferers

The biofeedback treatment given to tinnitus sufferers has in the main been directed at reduction of stress rather than at reducing the perception of or the noticeability or loudness of the tinnitus *per se*. House (1981b) reports finding tinnitus patients attending her clinic to be depressed, but that such individuals accept biofeedback more readily as a treatment than psychotherapy. The treatment regime implemented by House consisted of ten weekly one-hour sessions in which patents were taught to reduce their muscle activity (most commonly used because such muscles are already under voluntary control) and to increase their skin temperature. The technique was complemented by teaching the patients 'deep relaxation' exercises. Of the 132 patients who completed the training, 15 per cent were reported to be 'totally relieved', 29 per cent reported that they were 'very much improved', 33 per cent reported that they were 'improved enough to tolerate their tinnitus', and 23 per cent reported 'no change', but half of these said they now understood what made their tinnitus worse. None of the patients reported feeling worse after the treatment.

Elfner, May, Moore and Mendelson (1981) give a case-study report of a patient who exhibited 'the usual complaints of frustration, annoyance, and lack of sleep associated with tinnitus'. After two months of weekly biofeedback sessions in the clinic, together with training at home using a portable device to feedback skin temperature, the patient was reported to be relieved of the psychological symptoms associated with the tinnitus. A one-year follow-up demonstrated that the patient remained free of psychological symptoms although the subjective loudness of the tinnitus ringing was judged to be the same as at the onset of the tinnitus. This patient had been given instruction in reducing forehead muscle activity by electromyographic feedback as well as instructions on raising the temperature in an index finger. In the first month of treatment, apart from weekly clinic attendance, the patient practiced for half an hour each evening just before going to bed. After the second month of such training the patient was told to use the technique (without resort to equipment) whenever he felt tired or had trouble with the tinnitus. At the one-year follow-up the ringing did not bother the patient 'as long as he kept his mind off it', and this individual could still voluntarily raise the temperature of his finger.

Unfortunately, such case studies, though indicative and illustrative, do not confirm to the 'ground rules' for the effective evaluation of such treatment regimes. A sizeable number of individuals need to be treated successfully before general pronouncements can be made, and it must be clear that 'recovery' is not simply a function of time. Recovery must also be shown to be independent of the effects of the expectancy of relief — the *placebo effect*. New treatments should also be evaluated against a background of other available treatments; are they better, cheaper, simpler to administer? And the individual's condition should be assessed thoroughly and as objectively as possible before and after treatment, since many disorders treated by biofeedback may be *intermittently* troublesome. Finally, long-term follow-up is needed to examine what happens when the formal treatment is withdrawn and the individual is confronted with the stresses of his or her everyday life.

Some scepticism about the effects of biofeedback on individuals with tinnitus is raised by Galanos (1982), who notes that few studies include a control group of untreated patients and that many use relaxation training together with biofeedback methods, so it is impossible to see which technique is having the effect. He also suggests apparently positive success rates may reflect the type of individual motivated to be part of and continue with such a treatment regime — the ones on whom it may prove ineffective might tend not to be included as subjects in the study. He also points out that there is little evidence that ability to relax the forehead muscles, for example, generalises to other muscle groups (thus indicating a *general* relaxation element that is effective), and that some individuals might find outside help, personal attention, gadgetry and going to clinics useful, because it facilitates the *expectancy* of some positive result.

Nowhere does it appear to have been unequivocally demonstrated that biofeedback has an effect in lessening tinnitus or in helping individuals cope with the stress associated with it that is superior to more simple relaxation techniques.

RELAXATION TECHNIQUES

Relaxation techniques, like biofeedback techniques, if they are to be successful require time, dedication and effort. It may take many years for an individual to reach such a level of tension that a quite tangible expression of it, a heart attack perhaps, is the outcome. Years of *learning* to let a variety of essentially non-stressful stimuli make one tense cannot be undone in minutes — which is why relaxation techniques are not 'off the shelf panaceas' — they are not *instant* solutions. This in itself may present a problem. The tense, harassed individual may feel that 'having to do relaxation exercises' is yet another chore on the list of daily activities that, hard-pressed for time, he or she has nevertheless got to get through. Because individuals *habituate* to tension, get used to it as 'normal' and forget what relaxation used to be like (or turn to alcohol or other drugs to 'relax'), they may consider 'treatment' unnecessary until it is too late and the damage is done — when a concrete physical manifestation *does* appear. In this respect the tension suffered by many individuals with tinnitus may often be of a specific 'tension headache' variety, although this will in many cases overlay a more general level of bodily tension that might go unrecognised.

Being able to stand back and recognise tension before much damage is done can be quite difficult, and often friends and relatives see all too clearly signs of tension in an individual who cannot see them in him or herself. Many people with tinnitus do, of course, feel tense and recognise it, and many more may wonder what might help them cope with tinnitus better without necessarily having thought of 'relaxation' as a possibility. Many individuals equate relaxing with pursuing non-work activities, or with drinking alcohol or taking drugs, but this is not the relaxation to which relaxation techniques are directed — these are directed at bringing muscles more readily under conscious voluntary control, since many consider that by having a relaxed body it is possible to have a relaxed mind.

Most relaxation techniques ask the individual to set aside ten to 20 minutes, once or twice a day (in the morning before starting work, and at night before going to bed, perhaps), in a quiet room where there will be no interruptions. The person is usually advised to wear loose clothes, or at least untighten his or her belt, so that the stomach is unrestricted in deep breathing, and to lie on a carpeted floor with cushions under the neck and knees, if this is most comfortable, or to sit in a comfortable armchair with a high back to act as a headrest, or to sit crosslegged with his or her back to a wall. Some positions are more suitable for certain techniques. The individual may be asked to gaze at an object in direct view, or to close his or her eyes lightly.

Muscle relaxation techniques

Conventional relaxation techniques involve the subject listening to the therapist (or subsequently to a tape) giving instructions concerning the relaxation of various muscles in the body. Often subjects who are habitually tense or who have habituated to tension simply assume that a relaxed muscle is a slight variation on what they already have — namely a tense muscle — and directives simply to 'relax your neck muscles' may not work because the subject just cannot do it to order.

Perhaps the most widely used muscle relaxation technique is that of Jacobson, who in 1929 showed that strong emotional states like anxiety could be markedly inhibited if a person was in a state of deep relaxation. In Jacobson's many experiments, various indices concerning the autonomic nervous system, as well as self-reports, indicated that the anxiety of subjects was reduced after they had learned to 'let go' of their muscles through a progressive programme of contracting and relaxing muscle groups of the body. This technique, progressive relaxation, is widely used in regimes to desensitise people to things they find anxiety-making and it is demonstrably effective (Davison and Neale 1982). It is useful for habitually tense people because it enables them more readily to be consciously aware of muscular tension (rather than simply taking it for granted) and to be able to relax their muscles at will. Deep muscle relaxation is associated with deep mental relaxation and freedom from feelings of anxiety or stress and tension.

Usually *deep breathing* exercises are an integral part of progressive relaxation, deep breathing essentially also inducing a relaxed state, shallow breathing often being indicative of a tense one. The subject may at first be encouraged to concentrate on breathing, taking deep breaths, letting the stomach then the chest rise on inhalation through the nose, holding the breath for a short while, and then letting the breath out naturally, rather than forcing it out. The muscles may be attended to in individual detail or in larger muscle groupings. The therapist might start with the toes of one foot and ask the subject to contract them downwards as much as possible for a short while, then relax them, then tense them upwards as much as possible for a short while, then relax, while all the time breathing slowly and deeply. Then a similar technique will be used for the muscles of the foot, the calf, the thigh, etc. At first would-be relaxers usually find it difficult to follow instructions concerning muscle tensing and relaxing while at the same time maintaining regular slow deep breathing — the first thing the individual may do on being told to clench his or her fist might be to start to (unintentionally) hold the breath. Progressive relaxation tapes are usually very pleasant to listen to and easy to follow and a good family doctor would be able to recommend one.

COPING WITH TINNITUS STRESS — MISCELLANEOUS 'TREATMENT'

Yoga

Hatha yoga is concerned primarily with the physical aspect of one's being and comprises a series of body postures (asanas) and certain breathing exercises. Many of the final postures require weeks or months of progressive practice to maintain, so newcomers to yoga start with elementary positions rather than those final positions often publicised in connection with yoga. Most yoga sessions start with a deep relaxation posture (Savasana). There are many introductory books to Hatha yoga exercises and Hittleman's (1969) is easy to follow. Winter yoga evening classes are usually on offer by the local educational establishments of most towns and cities, and often provide a good introduction. As with other relaxation techniques, subjects are usually requested to carry on with exercises at home on a regular systematic daily basis. Tinnitus sufferers wondering what to do in the long winter evenings might be well advised to try yoga classes. Although yoga exercises might stretch the spine, spinal manipulation, particularly of the neck as in osteopathy or chiropractice is *not* a treatment to be advised, since it can sometimes make the tinnitus worse.

Hypnosis

Hypnosis is not likely to have much effect on tinnitus, which is a very 'hard' symptom, although it may be used as an adjunct to relaxation therapy. It is no more effective than relaxation exercises in most cases but often much more costly. Self-hypnosis is much akin to listening to tapes using suggestion and imagination techniques. Brattberg (1983) reports a study in which 32 patients with tinnitus were treated with hypnosis. Treatment consisted of a one-hour consultation with the physician followed by four weeks of daily home practice while listening to an audio-tape recording of approximately 15 minutes duration that had been made during the introductory one-hour session. The 15-minute tape used progressive relaxation techniques to induce the patient into a hypnotic trance. The hypnotherapy aim was to induce the patient into as relaxed a state as possible, thereafter implanting the suggestion that the patient would no longer be troubled by the noise. Brattberg concluded that the technique worked best with subjects who were most suggestible (as detected by an arm levitation test), and was least successful with patients who may also have some depression. Twenty-two of the 32 patients treated learned in one month 'to disregard the disturbing noise', which Brattberg suggests is a considerable gain in the ratio of therapy to time required. He goes on to suggest that this method of using a tape of a relaxation-hypnotherapy session at home is much less time-consuming than multiple visits to a therapist.

Acupuncture

Acupuncture is an ancient Chinese therapy in which fine needles are inserted into the skin at certain defined points on the body; this is thought to stimulate the 'chi' (the vital energy that runs through the body in channels called 'meridians'). The Medical Adviser to the British Tinnitus Association points out that he has received one or two accounts of acupuncture being of help but these were all in cases where the tinnitus was not continuous but was intermittent, so it was hard to tell if it was the acupuncture itself that had some effect. He also mentions having received hundreds of letters from people having had long courses of acupuncture costing them large sums of money that have been no help at all. Hansen, Hansen and Bentzen (1982) report a double-blind cross-over trial in which acupuncture treatment for tinnitus was given using the 'proper' acupuncture points in contrast to a placebo treatment that was given which did not use the proper acupuncture points. The study found no significant differences in effect between using the proper and other acupuncture points, although the tinnitus was generally rated as less pronounced during the course of the study. This effect was itself only significant in the group that received placebo acupuncture followed by genuine acupuncture. It is likely that these results can be explained in terms of general placebo effects.

Ultrasound

Sound that cannot usually be heard by individuals with normal hearing is often referred to as ultrasound. The ideal tinnitus masker would be a device that emitted a noise inaudible to the listener that had the effect of lessening the tinnitus or abolishing it altogether. Vernon (1981) reports, however, not being able to find masking sounds with such properties. Currently attempts are being made to investigate this possibility further. A device that transmits an inaudible high-frequency ultrasound through the mastoid bone to the inner ear is on trial, and anecdotal evidence to date suggests it can in some instances 'mask' the tinnitus without affecting hearing acuity (Kennedy 1984).

'Burn-out'

The rationale for 'burn-out' as a treatment for tinnitus is that if the tinnitus is of a sufficiently precise pitch it might be generated at a particular site in the cochlea, which is physically organised on a tone-responsive basis, low tones being responded to at the 'far' end (the apex) and high tones at the 'near' end. If the hair cells at this localised site could be put out of action by high-intensity noise of the same frequency, this might halt the tinnitus — or so the idea goes.

Young and Lowry (1983) report that one of the investigators had tinnitus of a high 10,000-Hz pitch equivalent in the left ear and no tinnitus in the right ear. The subject was exposed in the left ear to a steady tone of 2000 Hz pitch (in the high notes region of a piano) at quite a loud volume (107 dB SPL) for ten minutes. This exposure resulted in a *permanent* tinnitus in *both* ears of a pitch around 10,000 Hz, which fortunately was quite quiet. Other high-intensity stimulations of the left ear also produced different forms of short-term tinnitus in the right ear. These findings suggest that central brain processes may be mediating the effect of external noise and illustrate how permanent damage might easily result in 'burn-out' treatments.

Tinnitus inhibitors

One form of inhibitor is a small body-worn instrument produced by C.F. Kemp of Australia, which has been claimed to stop tinnitus. It produces a single tone of variable pitch and volume. It is claimed that by 'tuning in' to the tinnitus pitch you can get rid of it after only 30 seconds or so of exposure to noise of the same pitch from the inhibitor. Hazell (1982b) considers the instrument to be dangerous in so far as it can produce noise levels above those recommended in industry, and could thus be permanently damaging to the ear, despite claims in the instructions to the opposite.

Perhaps it is fitting that a chapter on 'Treatment and Therapies' should end with a warning about paying good money for ineffective treatments or instruments, or worse still for devices or therapies that might in the long-term prove to be actually damaging. Decisions made in *desperation* to pay for and try treatment, may well not prove to be wise decisions. Masking devices apart, perhaps the most effective and cheapest form of 'treatment' for tinnitus is sensible life-style management with learning of relaxation exercise for good measure. This, together with information and reassurance from professionals and fellow 'sufferers', may remain the mainstay of therapy for idiopathic tinnitus for some time to come (Hazell 1979b).

15

Tinnitus Maskers — Their Role in Tinnitus Management

Masking occurs when one sound is used to 'cover up or drown out' another sound. Masking of one sound by another is a common everyday experience. For example, road traffic noise or aircraft noise can easily mask speech. Speakers then have to choose either to shout above the noise or to pause until the noise subsides. Often, masking is by industrial machines that produce noise with a broad spectrum, i.e. containing a wide range of frequencies. However, significant masking can be produced by a sound with a narrowband spectrum, such as a tone, of moderate intensity. Usually, the masking sound 'covers up' the sound that we are trying to hear, but fortunately it can work the other way around. Speech or music and other sounds can be used to mask annoying sounds, such as buzzes, whines or a nearby conversation that may, on their own, be regarded as irritating and annoying. Music is often used to provide a pleasant working environment, and to cover up what otherwise might be a monotonous or irritating sound environment. Use of sound this way is certainly not a recent idea, and it is not too surprising that researchers and tinnitus sufferers have attempted to use masking to provide relief from tinnitus.

It has been claimed that a hearing aid, in those suffering from deafness and tinnitus, can be used for masking of tinnitus, since the restoration of hearing capability by the aid also results in the tinnitus being masked by the amplified external sounds. This does occur in many cases, and fitting a hearing aid to restore the hearing capability would be a sensible first step in attempting to relieve tinnitus. However, in many cases it is not possible to use amplified external sound to mask the tinnitus. For example, the frequency response of the hearing aid may be inadequate to amplify sound components in the high-frequency region to a level sufficient to produce masking of a high-frequency tinnitus. Also, the hearing loss of the sufferer may be too great for amplified external sounds to produce any perceptual effect. The tinnitus sufferer may have adequate hearing in the speech frequency range and amplification of sounds in this frequency region may be considered as more annoying than the tinnitus. Lastly, this type of masking depends on the presence of external sounds that may not always be on hand. For these reasons, it may be necessary to introduce noise specifically for the purpose of masking the tinnitus.

Combination hearing aid and tinnitus maskers do exist, but in its simplest form the tinnitus masker merely produces noise. Vernon (1977, 1981) was an early pioneer in this field and has striven to produce a tinnitus masker that could be 'tailored' to the individual tinnitus. The first maskers, however, produced a wideband noise in the mid-to-high frequency range, i.e. with frequency components in the range 500 to 4000 Hz. Early studies of tinnitus masking did produce encouraging results, in that provision of a masker often resulted in a reduction in the severity of the tinnitus symptoms, and for many sufferers it was claimed that the tinnitus symptoms could be managed and controlled by use of a tinnitus masker. In a proportion of sufferers using tinnitus maskers, the tinnitus was reported as reduced in intensity or completely absent after a period of masker use. This phenomena has been termed 'residual inhibition' by Vernon (see Chapter 5). Other encouraging results for tinnitus maskers have come from Hazell (1981). Before considering these results in more detail it is worth examining the underlying factors at play when masking is used to relieve and manage tinnitus.

WHY SHOULD MASKING WORK?

There are a number of reasons why masking might be expected to give some relief from tinnitus. Consider the tinnitus itself — it is a sound that has no external reference, it usually is unharmonious, monotonous and, apart from the fact of its capacity to intrude on the attention of the sufferer, it is uninteresting. Certainly, it is unwanted! The replacement or substitution of the tinnitus by another sound would not appear at first sight to improve matters, however the tinnitus-masking sound does have external reference, it can be modified in many ways, indeed complex masking sounds, such as music and speech, can be used, and perhaps more importantly, it can be switched off at will.

This ability to control the sound may be an important psychological factor. Glass and Singer (1972) showed that for subjects performing a moderately difficult task in the presence of noise, subjects who are given the option of controlling the presence or level of loud noise but who are asked only to modify the noise level if necessary will perform subsequent tasks better than a control group of subjects who are not given the option of control over noise levels. This is true even when it is arranged that both groups are subjected to the same level and duration of noise. Thus, one group has *perceived control* over the noise, while the other group has no control over the noise. Regarded in this way, the masking sound may seem more preferable than the tinnitus, since the masking noise can be manipulated but the tinnitus sufferer cannot exercise a similar level of control over the tinnitus. This would imply that user control of the masker, in terms of control of duration, level and frequency of use, is an important factor in the capacity of masking to relieve tinnitus.

One possible way in which tinnitus masking may operate is by analogy with 'scratching an itch'. That is, the irritating sound is swamped out by a more intense but more diffuse sound. However, such a mechanism, like scratching itself, is unlikely to provide lasting satisfaction. Another possibility is that the masking sound is more 'pleasant' than the tinnitus, since some sounds would always be preferable to others. In this case the choice is between continuous presence of one sound (the tinnitus) and continuous presence of the other sound (the tinnitus-masking sound). The tinnitus masker provides the sufferer with that choice, and as long as the tinnitus-masking sound is genuinely preferable to the tinnitus (or at least preferable for some substantial period of time) then tinnitus masking should be a useful treatment for the tinnitus.

Further examination of this idea of substitution of one sound for another suggests that two factors may be involved; the provision of (a) a sound that is easier to ignore than the tinnitus, and (b) a sound that is more pleasant to listen to than is the tinnitus. It may be that the design of tinnitus-masking sounds could try to optimise for one or both of these factors. For example, use of white noise that has been bandpass filtered to select a band of frequency components within the auditory range, *may* produce a sound that the subject finds easier to ignore than the tinnitus. The use of music or speech, on the other hand, would be an example of masking sounds that are less annoying or indeed welcomed by the subject.

Tinnitus maskers initially were designed foremost to drown out

the tinnitus by using broadband noise (noise with frequency components in the range 1 to 8 kHz). In order to increase the masking
power, attempts were made to produce 'tailored' noise. The primary
emphasis was to mask the tinnitus, although it was realised that the
tinnitus-masking noise should ideally only mask the tinnitus, and not
other external sounds that would be of interest, such as speech.
Controlled studies of the rated annoyance of sounds (see Kryter 1985
for a review) have shown that sounds can be arranged in terms of
their annoyance value. A recent study (Terry and Jones 1986) in
which both normal-hearing non-tinnitus subjects and tinnitus
subjects were used has suggested that noise bands of intermediate
bandwidth (i.e. a noise band that would occupy only about one-
quarter to one-half of the human auditory range rather than a wide-
band masker that covers the most of the range, say 100 Hz to 8 kHz)
would be rated as less annoying than other possible tinnitus-masking
sounds, such as wideband noise or pure tones.

Whatever the mechanism by which tinnitus masking provides
relief, a choice between alternative tinnitus maskers in terms of their
rated annoyance or sound preference values would appear to be
warranted (Letowski and Thompson 1985). The results from the
above studies would enable such a choice to be made and further
refinements of tinnitus maskers can be made with reference to these
factors.

DOES MASKING WORK?

Tinnitus masking can provide an effective relief from tinnitus for at
least some tinnitus sufferers for at least some of the time. However
the ability to predict which sufferers would benefit from the use of
maskers and by how much is a more difficult question to answer.
A recent review of masker effectiveness was made by McFadden
(1982). The review suggests that the following points may be made.
The early work on tinnitus was carried out by Jack Vernon and his
colleagues at their clinic in Oregon. Their procedure is to carry out
an audiological examination of the tinnitus sufferer, a process that
includes a test for residual inhibition. Following this, a decision is
made as to whether masking may give relief, and if this is considered
likely then a recommendation is made to try a hearing aid, tinnitus
masker or a combined aid/masker. The initial reports were
encouraging, with a figure of 72 per cent of those recommended for
treatment claiming relief from masking. However, it is difficult to

quantify the amount of relief. In a very few exceptional cases it has been claimed that following a period of masking the tinnitus disappeared completely and has not returned (an interval now of several years, assuming the tinnitus has not re-occurred). More commonly, a period of 35 to 40 minutes during which the tinnitus cannot be heard is reported by the sufferer after one day's use of the masker. Relief also occurs while the masker is on as long as the sufferer rates the masker noise as less annoying or distracting than the tinnitus. There have been improvements in tailoring the masking noise to the specific tinnitus, and a re-evaluation of the probabilities of obtaining relief through masking, using the Oregon data, indicates that (a) masking does contribute some relief (complete or partial — complete relief is less common than partial) for about 56 per cent of those for whom a masker recommendation (aid and/or masker) is made, and (b) given that you have tinnitus, there is about a 42 per cent chance that masking will provide some relief.

Recently more data on masker use and effectiveness has been reported. A large scale clinical trial of tinnitus maskers has just been completed. The trial was conducted at three different centres (University College Hospital; the Royal National Throat, Ear and Nose Hospital and the General Hospital of Nottingham) and investigated the effect of tinnitus counselling and the benefit of tinnitus maskers (Hazell et al. 1985). In this study comparisons can be made of groups of tinnitus sufferers who received counselling and were fitted with maskers, and a group who received counselling but were not given maskers. The trial lasted six months and the subjects were given questionnaires at the beginning and at three-month intervals. Hearing tests and psychoacoustical tests designed to evaluate the tinnitus were given before and after the trial. The basic results suggested that maskers were beneficial, although the amount of benefit was not outstanding if the counselled non-masker and masker groups were compared. This was a large and important study and it would be difficult to evaluate thoroughly the results in a small space. However, let us briefly summarise the findings and examine the claims proposed for the beneficial effects of using tinnitus maskers. The main results were as follows:

1. Counselling is of help
2. Further benefit is given by use of masking instruments
3. Maskers are often more effective than hearing aids
4. There is no evidence of any harmful effect of masking
5. None of the currently employed audiometric or tinnitus tests can

191

be regarded as predictive, either of severity of tinnitus or of the eventual outcome of masker therapy. However, certain measurements may help as a guide to management of patients.

Tests of hearing were carried out before and after the masker trial and there was no evidence of any harmful effect of masking. The method of assessing the effect of masking on the tinnitus was by questionnaire. One of the questions posed was 'While wearing the instrument does it help to mask the tinnitus?' The subject was asked to select one of the following replies:

1. All the time
2. Three-quarters of the time
3. Half the time
4. One-quarter of the time
5. Never

The range of questions asked covered most aspects of masker usage and the effects of the masker on the tinnitus. The results suggested a general overall benefit of wearing the masker. However, there is always a bias towards favourable response since most subjects tend to be slightly generous in their response for fear of appearing ungrateful for the time and effort spent in fitting the masker. It is difficult to avoid problems of this kind when attempting to assess a subjective symptom (in most cases) such as tinnitus and it is desirable to have alternative methods of evaluation when possible.

A second method of evaluating changes in the tinnitus was by means of tinnitus psychophysical measurements, i.e. loudness balance, maskability and residual inhibition (RI). The best possible result would be a significant measure from the questionnaire indicating reduced severity of the tinnitus, and less anxiety about the condition, coupled with data from the psychophysical tests showing lower loudness levels, increased maskability and maybe increased amounts of RI; in the control groups, tinnitus measures should indicate no or little change.

It is perhaps unfortunate that not all centres had a control group. However, the ethical considerations of providing no treatment for those seeking help may have ruled out this option. Another factor is the amount of additional counselling the masker and hearing aid groups received due to masker fitting, plus the interview in which the masker effectiveness questionnaire was given. This 'extra attention' may have contributed to the difference between groups. The actual findings do show some significant differences between the masker and non-masker groups, but the psychophysical tests show no significant improvement in the tinnitus after long-term masker usage.

It may be that for some individuals, tinnitus maskers are of great benefit in the management of tinnitus (for example those showing residual inhibition for significant periods) but it appears to be accepted that the main role of masking is to control tinnitus rather than to produce a cure.

There does seem to be evidence from this study that in patients with hearing difficulties, maskers are more effective than hearing aids in relieving tinnitus. This finding is highlighted in the companion paper by Stephens and Corcoran (1985). Interestingly, these authors conclude that for patients with little or no hearing difficulty, masking is no more effective than limited counselling. The psychophysical measures of tinnitus do not appear to reveal much information with regard to predicting the effect of masking. It is likely that more extensive tests are required.

The three-centre study has been extremely valuable in the evaluation of tinnitus maskers, but clearly further research is required to identify those tinnitus sufferers most likely to benefit from masking.

ARE SOME FORMS OF TINNITUS UNMASKABLE?

The answer to this question is undoubtedly yes. On the one hand there are cases of tinnitus sufferers in whom the hearing loss is so great that sounds, no matter how intense, cannot produce a sensation. In this situation masking cannot occur. On the other hand, in cases in whom the tinnitus is of low intensity and the hearing ability is near normal, then the tinnitus is very easily masked by low-level sounds. It is possible to have tinnitus that is masked very easily by tones of any frequency within the audiometric range (see Chapter 5). In other types of tinnitus the frequency of the tone masker or the spectral composition of the noise masker determine whether the tinnitus will be masked. There are also types of tinnitus in which the masker produces an intense sensation, but in which the tinnitus remains unmasked. In some cases, the lack of masking may be because the tinnitus is made up of many components, and the masker is not tailored (spectrally shaped) to cover or mask all the components of the tinnitus. In other cases, the masker may have to be applied to both ears before the tinnitus is masked. Sufficient attention to the structure and manner of presentation of the masker will increase the percentage of tinnitus cases that can be masked, however there will always be cases in whom the tinnitus cannot be masked.

These cases of unmaskability may be divided into two general categories: (1) Those in whom the hearing loss is too great for the tinnitus masker to produce sufficient sensation in the frequency region of the tinnitus. (2) Those in whom there appears to be sufficient hearing ability but where no tinnitus masker can mask the tinnitus.

In the second category, the lack of masking may suggest a central or high-level site for the tinnitus. It is possible that the tinnitus modulates the incoming peripheral signal so that some aspect of the tinnitus is present no matter what the auditory input. For these cases tinnitus masking cannot provide relief although the lack of response may be of some diagnostic use to the clinician. However, even when masking is not an option, it is always possible that, where there is hearing ability, a sound stimulus, such as music, may work to distract attention from the tinnitus.

RESIDUAL INHIBITION

So far the benefit of masking has largely been discussed in terms of a possible relief from tinnitus obtained in the presence of the masking sound. However, it has been found that benefits can occur in the period following use of the masker. The tinnitus is often reported to be reduced and even absent for substantial periods following masker usage. This phenomenon has been termed residual inhibition (RI) and was discussed in Chapter 5. The discussion in this chapter will be concerned with the amount of RI that might be expected from the use of tinnitus maskers. RI is obviously of great interest because if the periods of RI could be lengthened, an effective 'remedy' for some types of tinnitus would be at hand.

The relevant questions concerning RI are:

1. Does RI inevitably follow masking?
2. What period of RI can be expected?
3. Is it possible to produce ever-increasing amounts of RI?
4. What is the mechanism or mechanisms that are involved?

194

The answers to these questions, however, are not yet fully available and more basic research is required. It is known that RI can be readily induced in a substantial fraction of tinnitus sufferers (estimates vary depending on sources, but from about one-third to one-half of tinnitus sufferers). However, it is necessary to make sure that the tinnitus is masked when assessing whether RI is present.

It has been shown that the amount of RI induced will vary, depending on the composition of the masker, and that duration, intensity, bandwidth and centre frequency of the tinnitus masker are important determinants of the amount of RI produced (Feldmann 1971, Vernon 1977, Terry *et al.* 1983). Not all tinnitus maskers are equivalent in producing RI. Because RI depends on masker duration and intensity, tests for RI should be made with masker durations of at least one minute and the intensity of the masker should be at least 10 dB SPL above the level required to mask the tinnitus (Evered and Lawrenson 1981, Terry *et al.* 1983). If the dBA value of the masker that masks the tinnitus is below 60 dBA, it may be necessary to use a masker in the range 70 to 90 dBA in order to induce RI. Where short masker durations are used, e.g. 60 secs, reduced tinnitus loudness might typically be expected to last over a period of one to three minutes. In one experimental study, an increase in masker duration (one to ten minutes) did in general increase the period of RI, however the increase was smaller than a proportional increase and was more nearly logarithmically related to masker duration (Terry *et al.* 1983). However in other studies in which a larger selection of tinnitus sufferers have been tested, quite substantial periods of RI have been reported (Vernon and Meikle 1981). In some cases the RI has lasted a matter of days and longer.

The amount of RI may differ between tinnitus types. The tinnitus that is associated with sensorineural loss, which often results from industrial noise exposure, appears to show significant amounts of RI. Although the amount of RI is often not sufficient to be of real clinical use, it is often of great psychological importance to demonstrate to the tinnitus sufferer that the tinnitus can be altered, even if only for a short time.

The actual mechanism underlying RI is unclear. Masking the tinnitus does not inevitably lead to RI. The masker may act as:

1. An input of energy into a damaged system. An analogy may be a knock to restore a loose connection, as in a faulty radio set, although this is unlikely to be the method by which a masker produces RI. The energy might also temporarily alter the local

biomechanical or biochemical environment in the area producing the tinnitus.

2. A stimulus causing some fatigue or adaptation in some area of the system that was previously responding to the tinnitus.

The intensity of masking sounds required to produce RI are often sufficiently strong to produce temporary threshold shifts in the tinnitus frequency region. This finding may link with point (2) but it also brings up the possibility that uncontrolled use of a masker may, in fact, cause more damage to the hearing system; a fact that has been appreciated by workers and clinicians in this field but which nevertheless needs emphasising.

CHOOSING A TINNITUS MASKER

There are a number of maskers currently available and they vary both in the spectral composition of the noise-masking stimulus and the ability to vary or tune the masking stimulus. The main characteristics (e.g. spectral composition and output level) of some of the currently available maskers are shown in an appendix to this chapter. The choice of the correct masker for the individual depends on a number of factors, including cost. A recommendation from the ENT clinic is advised but any masker should be obtained on a trial basis first. The features to look and listen for are, first, the volume control: can the intensity of the masker be changed easily? Is there sufficient volume to mask the tinnitus? If masking only occurs at maximum volume then it is possible that the spectral composition of the noise masker may require adjustment. Is there such a control (e.g. like a bass or treble control on a hi-fidelity amplifier or radio) on the masker? This control should be adjusted together with the volume control to produce a masking noise that will mask the tinnitus at the lowest masker intensity.

Photographs of some commonly available maskers are shown in Figure 15.1.

Another possible masking system would be a portable tape-recorder with a noise-masking sound recorded onto tape. There now exist high-fidelity tape recorders with stereo headphones that can be carried in the pocket. The advantage of this system is that a tailored noise masker, specific for the individual tinnitus, can be recorded onto tape. This could be done after an audiological examination in the laboratory. It should be emphasised that these tape recorders are quite powerful and can produce high sound levels at the ear, so that prolonged use at high output levels would invariably cause hearing damage. Their use would therefore need to be supervised and as a general principle the volume controls should be set to the minimum required for masking the tinnitus.

For tinnitus that has a high pitch and that stems from a high-frequency region, the most effective masker is likely to be the one with relatively more power in the mid-to-high spectral region. Conversely, a low-pitched tinnitus would be more easily masked by a noise masker that had a concentration of power in the mid-to-low frequency region. If a noise masker had equal power throughout the audiometric frequency range, then although this masker could be used to mask both high and low pitched tinnitus, it would be an inefficient masker and would have to be relatively more intense than a tailored masker and would consequently be rated as louder and probably more annoying than a tailored masker. There is, however, a need for caution when using noise bands that are constructed with steep slopes or skirts (i.e. the rate at which energy reduces as frequency changes at the edges of the noise bands, usually specified in terms of dB/octave). Noise bands with very steep slopes (> 200 dB/octave) are known to produce audible after-effects often after only short exposure times, and it is possible that such masking noises may themselves constitute a danger of producing tinnitus (McFadden and Pasanen 1980).

WHEN TO MASK AND FOR HOW LONG?

The question of when to mask depends almost entirely upon the individual but the duration of the masking session should be regulated. A large number of tinnitus cases arise in association with noise-induced hearing damage and there would be little value in increasing the amount of hearing damage by over-zealous use of tinnitus maskers. Some users may have the idea of using the masker to 'burn out' or eradicate that part of the system that is producing the tinnitus. Unfortunately this would be very difficult to do, even by using carefully designed sound stimuli, and there is no guarantee that the tinnitus would not be made worse. There are standards of noise exposure that have been designed to reduce the risk of noise-induced hearing damage. These standards are called damage risk criteria and are shown in the table 15.1 below. Impulsive or transient sounds are more damaging than continuous sounds, and tonal or narrowband are more damaging than continuous sounds, and tonal

Figure 15.1: Photographs of tinnitus maskers

a)

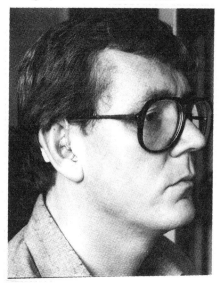

or narrow band are more damaging than sounds that have a wideband spectrum. The maximum output of the masker should be known (in dB SPL and also in dBA) by the user and the amount of exposure to a noise masker for a given masker duration should be less than levels shown below.

Table 15.1: Damage risk criteria

Duration of continuous noise exposure	dBA
4 hours	93
2 hours	96
1 hour	99
30 minutes	102
15 minutes	105
7 minutes	108
4 minutes	111
2 minutes	114
1 minute	117

This table indicates risk criteria for industrial working conditions. It should be noted that the longer the exposure, the lower the criterion level, and that continuous 24-hour exposure may mean that levels below 70 or 60 dBA may be required to prevent damage. The minimum level to produce sufficient masking of the tinnitus should be the guideline and the maximum daily duration should be derived from this level. If very high levels are required to produce masking

b)

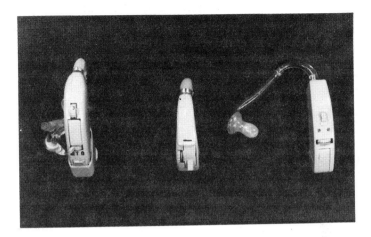

c)

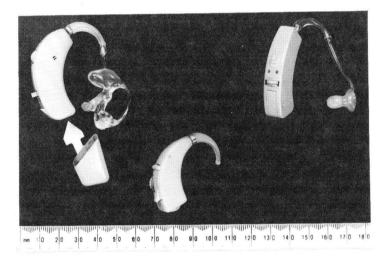

(a) A Danavox 105DV hearing-aid with 109W masker attachment and a 'non-occluding' or open-mould earpiece — worn behind the ear. (b) Danavox 105DV hearing aid/masker combination instrument; Tinnitus masker manufactured by P.C. Werth, model VTM1; a Starkey model TM3 tinnitus masker with a temporary earpiece.
(c) As (b) but showing the Danavox masker unit separated from the hearing aid.

199

then the maximum daily use of the masker may be restricted to very short periods. However, advice on this matter should be sought from the ENT clinic issuing the masker, where account will be taken of the nature and extent of any associated hearing loss and of the severity of the tinnitus. The clinic will also be able to monitor the effects of using the tinnitus masker.

One finding of interest with respect to masker duration is reported by Penner (1983), which may apply to a significant fraction of tinnitus sufferers, is that, unlike an external sound, the tinnitus masker level may have to be increased during presentation in order to keep the tinnitus masked. Penner found with some tinnitus subjects that, for masker presentations greater than five minutes, the tinnitus reappeared unless the masker level was correspondingly increased. The user of a masker may therefore need to exercise some caution and guard against any tendency to continually adjust the volume control upwards. Fortunately, the recent masker trial by Hazell *et al.* (1985) indicates that normal usage of the commonly available tinnitus maskers (e.g. Viennatone masker and the Danavox combination masker) are unlikely to produce damage to the hearing system.

As technology advances it will be possible to produce tailored noise maskers to suit the individual and which the individual can control (or even to synthesise tinnitus maskers to cater for any variation in the tinnitus).

Appendix

Characteristics of Currently Available Tinnitus Maskers

	Manufacturer	Model	Type	Tone Control	Noise Spectrum Hz	Output dB SPL	Battery type	Current mA
Behind the ear	P.C. Werth	VTM1	masker	yes	200–1000	87	SP 675	0.8
	Starkey	TM3	masker	user preset	variable	81/94	RM 675	0.85
	Danavox	775 V-TM	masker/aid	yes	100–20,000	105	RM 675	1.45
In the ear	P.C. Werth	EMTM4	masker	yes	variable	variable	RM 13	variable
	Starkey	TM3	masker	user preset	variable	81/94	RM 675	0.85
	G. Williams	Ear-canal	masker	no	medium band centred at 2000	87/112 (dB A)	●	●
Bedside masker	P.C. Werth	Sleep-a-tone	masker	yes	200–15,000 Hz	110	gv	●
	G. Williams	Bedside	masker	no	1000–6500	free field	MN 1604	●

● value not known

Note: Adapted from an article in British Tinnitus Association Newsletter

Manufacturers' addresses:

Williams Hearing Aid Services
Old Mill
23 Greenwich High Road
Greenwich
London SE10 8JL

Starkey Labs Ltd.
55–57 Wilmslow Road
Hadforth
Cheshire
SK9 3JJ

P.C. Werth
17 Stratford Place
London
W1N ODH

Danavox (GB) Ltd.
1 Cheyne Walk
Northampton

Epilogue

Future Developments

To date there is no simple effective remedy for tinnitus, although it can be said that the treatment of tinnitus today as offered by a modern tinnitus clinic has greatly improved. Current research into possible treatments of tinnitus is being undertaken on a number of fronts: in particular those of drug treatment, tinnitus masking and electrical suppression. The search for an effective drug remedy already has considerable momentum and a great deal is known of the effects of many drugs on the cochlea. The ideal drug would be taken orally and would suppress the tinnitus for some considerable time yet produce minimal side effects. Although no such drug is currently available, it is quite feasible that a suitable drug may be found. However, before trying any new drug tinnitus sufferers should seek advice from their local tinnitus clinic and consider very carefully the possible factors of drug dependency and side effects on both the hearing system and also on other physiological processes.

Research also continues on the development and use of tinnitus maskers in the role of tinnitus management. For example, Coles (1986) describes the use of a new 'in-the-ear' or ear-canal masker (manufacturer G. Williams, ear-canal masker, see appendix to Chapter 15). One advantage of this masker is that it may be worn at night and so aid sleep. It may also be considered more acceptable from a cosmetic point of view than a 'behind-the-ear' masker. A disadvantage is that it may block out too much of the external sound environment. In general, however, the design of tinnitus maskers and the flexibility and control over masker spectral content will continue to improve, together hopefully with a reduction in their cost.

Early work by Grapengiesser (1801), soon after Volta's (1800) invention of the battery, had suggested that DC current could suppress tinnitus, unfortunately the treatment also induced nausea. More recent work (Graham and Hazell 1976, Portman *et al.* 1979) has suggested that electrical stimulation could prove effective.

Vernon (1985) has summarised the research on recent attempts to produce electrical suppression of tinnitus. He discusses the work by Aran who, while involved with research on cochlear implants for hearing loss, discovered that an electrode on the round window could produce suppression of tinnitus if positive (anodal) stimulation was applied (Aran 1981, Aran and Cazals 1981, and Aran 1984). In this work pulsed stimulation was found to be the most effective, producing suppression of tinnitus in 60 per cent of cases tested. Chouard (1981), using electrodes placed on the skin close to the ear, also demonstrated tinnitus suppression, which in some cases lasted long after the period of stimulation, in a similar fashion to masking and residual inhibition. Vernon repeated Chouard's work, in particular testing a special electrical wave-form designed to produce the least possible tissue damage, with basically similar results. Shulman (1985) has also carried out research into tinnitus control using external electrical stimulation. The differing degrees of success in producing tinnitus suppression in these studies has led Vernon to speculate that control of the current path is perhaps the most important variable. Future research may well enable the safe effective placement of an electrode in or around the cochlea that could be used to control tinnitus.

Besides electrical suppression other possibilities exist. For example, there have been claims that ultrasound (very high frequency sound that cannot be heard) can produce residual inhibition or modify the tinnitus. Such a finding would be of great interest, since it would allow control over the tinnitus without an audible masker. However, whether ultrasound can modify tinnitus without producing side effects is a matter for research.

Apart from specific research on tinnitus, basic research into hearing and into the causes of deafness will also provide information on the possible mechanisms underlying tinnitus. Since tinnitus may arise in several ways, it is unlikely that a sudden 'cure' will be found for all cases of tinnitus, however it is perhaps not too optimistic to expect a gradual improvement in methods of control and management of tinnitus.

References Cited in the Text

Anon (1979) 'Tinnitus' (Editorial), *Lancet, 1* (8126), 1124

Aran, J.M. and Cazals, Y. (1981) 'Electrical suppression of tinnitus' in Ciba Foundation Symposium 85, *Tinnitus*, Pitman, London, pp. 217–31

Barrs, D.M. and Brackmann, D.E. (1984) 'Translabyrinthine Nerve Section: Effect on Tinnitus', *Journal of Laryngology and Otology*, Supplement No. 9, Proceedings of the 2nd International Tinnitus Seminar, New York, 10 and 11 June 1983, pp. 287–93

Batteau, D.W. (1967) 'The Role of the Pinna in Human Localization', *Proceedings Royal Society London Series B, 168*, 158–80

von Bekesy, G. (1928) 'Zur Theorie des Horens: Die Schwingungsform der Basilarmembrane', *Physik. Zeits., 29*, 793–810

von Bekesy, G. (1960) *Experiments in hearing*, Wiley, New York

Brama, I. and Fainaru, M. (1980) 'Inner Ear Involvement in Behçet's Disease', *Archives of Otolaryngology, 106* (4), 215–7

Brattberg, G. (1983) 'An Alternative Method of Treating Tinnitus: Relaxation-Hypnotherapy Primarily Through the Home Use of a Recorded Audio Cassette', *International Journal of Experimental and Clinical Hypnosis, 31* (2), 90–7

Brennan, F.J. and Salerno, T.A. (1981) 'Surgical Treatment of Symptomatic Venous Hum', *Journal of Thoracic and Cardiovascular Surgery, 81* (1), 135–6

British Tinnitus Association (1980) 'Tinnitus Questions and Answers', *British Tinnitus Association Newsletter*, No. 7, i–vii

British Tinnitus Association (1984) 'Letters to the Editor', *British Tinnitus Association Newsletter*, No. 23, 12

Brookes, G.B., Maw, A.R. and Coleman, M.J. (1980) 'Costen's Syndrome — Correlation or Coincidence: A Review of 45 Patients with Temporomandibular Joint Dysfunction, Otalgia and Other Aural Symptoms', *Clinical Otolaryngology, 5* (1), 23–36

Brown, R.D., Penny, J.E., Henley, C.M., Hodges, K.B., Kupetz, S.A., Glenn, D.W. and Jobe, J.C. (1981) 'Ototoxic Drugs and Noise' in Ciba Foundation Symposium 85, *Tinnitus*, Pitman, London, pp. 151–71

Cathcart, J.M. (1982) 'Assessment of the Value of Tocainide Hydrochloride in the Treatment of Tinnitus', *Journal of Laryngology and Otology, 96* (11), 981–4

Chandler, J.R. (1983) 'Diagnosis and Cure of Venous Hum Tinnitus', *Laryngoscope, 93* (7), 892–5

Coles, R.R.A. (1981) 'Population Studies of Tinnitus', *British Tinnitus Association Newsletter*, No. 10, i–iv

Coles, R.R.A. (1983) 'Tinnitus Work in the Institute of Hearing Research', *British Tinnitus Association Newsletter*, No. 22, 2–6

Coles, R.R.A. (1984a) 'Epidemiology of Tinnitus: (2) Demographic and Clinical Features', *Journal of Laryngology and Otology*, Supplement No. 9, Proceedings of the 2nd International Tinnitus Seminar, New York, 10 and 11 June, 1983, pp. 195–202

Coles, R.R.A. (1984b) 'Epidemiology of Tinnitus: (1) Prevalence', *Journal of Laryngology and Otology*, Supplement No. 9, Proceedings of the 2nd International Tinnitus Seminar, New York, 10 and 11 June, 1983, pp. 7–15

Coles, R.R.A. (1986) 'The Williams Ear-canal Tinnitus Masker', *Sound-barrier*, No. 9, 17

Coles, R.R.A., Davis, A.C. and Haggard, M.P. (1981) 'Epidemiology of Tinnitus' in Ciba Foundation Symposium 85, *Tinnitus*, Pitman, London, pp. 16–34

Collard, M.E., Wagner, C.A. and Tingwald, F.R. (1982) 'Conditioned Middle Ear Muscle Tinnitus', *Annals of Otology Rhinology and Laryngology*, *91*, (3 part 1), 330–1

Daneshmend, T.K. (1979) 'Treatment of Tinnitus' (Letter), *British Medical Journal, 1* (6178), 1628

Davison, G.C. and Neale, J.M. (1982) *Abnormal psychology* (3rd edn), Wiley, New York

Dohlman, G.F. (1980) 'Mechanism of the Menière attack' *Journal of Oto-Rhino-Laryngology, 42*, 10–19

Donaldson, I. (1978) 'Tinnitus: A Theoretical View and a Therapeutic Study using Amylobarbitone', *Journal of Laryngology and Otology, 92* (2), 123–30

Donaldson, I. (1981) 'Tegretol: A Double Blind Trial in Tinnitus', *Journal of Laryngology and Otology, 95* (9), 947–51

Douek, E. (1981) 'Classification of Tinnitus' in Ciba Foundation Symposium 85, *Tinnitus*, Pitman, London, pp. 4–15

Douek, E. and Reid, J. (1968) 'The diagnostic value of tinnitus pitch' *Journal of Laryngology and Otology, 82*, 1039–42

Eggermont, J.J. (1984) 'Tinnitus: Some Thought About Its Origin', *Journal of Laryngology and Otology*, Supplement No. 9, Proceedings of the 2nd International Tinnitus Seminar, New York, 10 and 11 June, 1983, pp. 31–37

Ehrenberger, K. and Brix, R. (1983) 'Glutamic Acid and Glutamic Acid Diethylester in Tinnitus Treatment', *Acta Otolaryngologica, 95* (5–6), 599–605

Elfner, L.F., May, J.G., Moore, J.D. and Mendelson, J.M. (1981) 'Effects of EMG and Thermal Feedback Training on Tinnitus: A Case Study', *Biofeedback and Self-Regulation, 6* (4), 517–21

Evans, E.F. (1981a) 'Chairman's Introduction', in Ciba Foundation Symposium 85, *Tinnitus*, Pitman, London, pp. 1–3

Evans, E.F. (1981b) 'Chairman's Closing Remarks', in Ciba Foundation Symposium 85, *Tinnitus*, Pitman, London, pp. 295–9

Evans, E.F., Wilson, J.P. and Borerwe, T.A. (1981) 'Animal Models of Tinnitus' in Ciba Foundation Symposium 85, *Tinnitus*, Pitman, London, pp. 108–38

Evered, D. and Lawrenson, G. (1981) Ciba Symposium 85, *Tinnitus*, Pitman, London

Feldman, A.S. (1975) 'Acoustic-impedance measurements' in L.J. Bradford (ed.) *Physiological measures in the audio-vestibular system*, Academic Press, New York

Feldmann, H. (1971) 'Homolateral and Contralateral Masking of Tinnitus by Noise-Bands and by Pure Tones', *Audiology, 10* (3), 138–44

Feldmann, H. (1983) 'Time Patterns and Related Parameters in Masking of Tinnitus', *Acta Otolaryngologica, 95* (5–6), 594–8

Fernandez, A.O. (1983) 'Objective Tinnitus: A Case Report', *American Journal of Otology, 4* (4), 312–14

Fletcher, H., (1940) 'Auditory Patterns', *Review of Modern Physics, 12,* 47–65

Fowler, E.P. (1942) 'The "Illusion of loudness" of tinnitus: its aetiology and treatment', *Laryngoscope, 52,* 275–85

Frew, I.J.C. and Menon G.N. (1976) 'Betahistine hydrochloride in Menière's disease', *Postgraduate Medical Journal, 52,* 501–3

Galanos, A.N. (1982) 'Efficacy of Biofeedback in the Treatment of Tinnitus: Some Considerations (Letter)', *Southern Medical Journal, 75* (11), 1433

Gardner, G. (1984) 'Neurotolgic Surgery and Tinnitus', *Journal of Laryngology and Otology,* Supplement No. 9, Proceedings of the 2nd International Tinnitus Seminar, New York, 10 and 11 June, 1983, pp. 311–318

George, B., Reizine, D., Laurian, C., Riche, M.C. and Merland, J.J. (1983) 'Tinnitus of Venous Origin, Surgical Treatment by the Ligation of the Jugular Vein and Lateral Sinus Jugular Vein Anastomosis', *Journal of Neuroradiology, 10* (1), 23–30

Ghosh, P. (1978) 'Tinnitus: Classification and Acoustics', *Ear, Nose and Throat Journal, 57* (11), 504–9

Glanville, J.D., Coles, R.R.A. and Sullivan, B.M. (1971) 'A Family with High-tonal Objective Tinnitus', *Journal of Laryngology and Otology, 85,* 1–10

Glass, D.C. and Singer, J.E. (1972) 'Behavioral after-effects of unpredictable and uncontrollable aversive events', *American Scientist, 60,* 457–65

Glass, R.M. (1981) 'Ejaculatory Impairment from both Phenelzin and Imipramine, with Tinnitus from Phenelzine', *Journal of Clinical Psychopharmacology, 1* (3), 152–4

Golden, R.N., Evans, D.L. and Nau, C.H. (1983) 'Doxepin and Tinnitus', *Southern Medical Journal, 76* (9), 1204–5

Goodey, R.J. (1981) 'Drugs in the Treatment of Tinnitus' in Ciba Foundation Symposium 85, *Tinnitus,* Pitman, London, pp. 263–78

Goodhill, V. (1981) 'Ben H. Senturia Lecture. Leaking Labyrinth Lesions, Deafness, Tinnitus and Dizziness', *Annals of Otology Rhinology and Laryngology, 90* (2 Pt. 1), 99–106

Goodwin, P.E. and Johnson, R.M. (1980) 'The Loudness of Tinnitus', *Acta Otolaryngologica, 90* (5/6), 353–9

Graham, J. (1981) 'Paediatric Tinnitus', *Journal of Laryngology and Otology (Supplement 4),* 117–20

Graham, J.M. and Hazell, J.W.P. (1977) 'Electrical stimulation of the human cochlea using a transtympanic electrode', *British Journal of Audiology, 11,* 59–62

Grapengiesser, C.J.C. (1801) *Versuche den Galvanismus zur Heilung einiger Krankheiten anzuwenden,* Berlin, in der Myliussischen Buchhandlung

Green, R.J. (1976) *Tinnitus: Inhibition and Personality Characteristics,* Unpublished M.Sc Dissertation, University of Salford

Grover, B. (1984) 'Do You Suffer from Sociacusis?', *Soundbarrier* — Journal of the Royal National Institute for the Deaf, No. 1, 18

Hallam, R., Rachman, S. and Hinchcliffe, R. (1984) 'Psychological Aspects of Tinnitus' in S. Rachman (ed.), *Contributions to medical psychology*, Vol. 3, Pergamon Press, Oxford, pp. 31–53

Hansen, P.E., Hansen, J.H. and Bentzen, P. (1982) 'Acupuncture Treatment of Chronic Unilateral Tinnitus — A Double-blind Cross-Over Trial', *Clinical Otolaryngology*, 7 (5), 325–9

Hardison, J.E., Smith, R.B. 3rd, Crawley, I.S. and Battey, L.L. (1981) 'Self-heard Venous Hums', *Journal of the American Medical Association*, 245 (11), 1146–7

Hazell, J.W.P. (1979a) 'Tinnitus', *British Journal of Hospital Medicine*, 22 (5), 468–71

Hazell, J.W.P. (1979b) 'Tinnitus' in J. Ballantyne and J. Groves (eds.), *Scott-Brown's Disease of the Ear, Nose and Throat* (4th Edn), Butterworths, London, pp. 81–91

Hazell, J.W.P. (1979c) 'Tinnitus Research at the RNID 1974–1979', *British Tinnitus Association Newsletter*, No. 3, vi–viii

Hazell, J.W.P. (1980) 'Drug Treatment in Tinnitus: The Present Position', *British Tinnitus Association Newsletter*, No. 5, i–ii

Hazell, J.W.P. (1981a) 'Tinnitus', *The Practitioner*, 225 (1361), 1577–85

Hazell, J.W.P. (1981b) 'Patterns of Tinnitus: Medical Audiological Findings', *Journal of Laryngology and Otology* (Supplement 4), 39–47

Hazell, J.W.P. (1981c) 'Measurement of Tinnitus in Humans' in Ciba Foundation Symposium 85, *Tinnitus*, Pitman, London, pp. 35–48

Hazell, J.W.P. (1982a) 'Menière's Disease', *British Tinnitus Association Newsletter*, No. 16, i–iii

Hazell, J.W.P. (1982b) 'Tinnitus Inhibitor', *British Tinnitus Association Newsletter*, No. 18, iii–iv

Hazell, J.W.P. (1983) 'Flying and the Ear', *British Tinnitus Association Newsletter*, No. 19, ii–iii

Hazell, J.W.P. (1984) 'Future Research Possibilities', *British Tinnitus Association Newsletter*, No. 23, 6

Hazell, J.W.P. and Wood, S. (1981) 'Tinnitus Masking — A Significant Contribution to Tinnitus Management', *British Journal of Audiology*, 15 (4), 223–30

Hazell, J.W.P., Wood, S.M., Cooper, H.R., Stephens, S.D.G., Corcoran, A.L., Coles, R.R.A., Baskill, J.L. and Sheldrake, J.B. (1985) 'A clinical study of tinnitus maskers', *British Journal of Audiology 19*, 65–146

Heller, M.F. and Bergman, M. (1953) 'Tinnitus Aurium in Normally Hearing Persons', *American Otological Society Transactions*, 62, 73–83

Hinchcliffe, R. (1961) 'Prevalence of the Commoner Ear, Nose and Throat Conditions in the Adult Rural Population of Great Britain', *British Journal of Preventative and Social Medicine*, 15, 128–40

Hirsh, I.J. and Ward, W.D. (1952) 'Recovery of the auditory threshold after strong acoustic stimulation', *Journal of the Acoustical Society of America*, 24, 131–41

Hittleman, R. (1969) *Introduction to Yoga*, Bantam Books, New York

House, J.W. (1981a) 'Management of the Tinnitus Patient', *Annals of Otology Rhinology and Laryngology*, 90 (6 Pt. 1), 597–601

House, J.W. and Brackmann, D.E. (1981) 'Tinnitus: Surgical Treatment' in Ciba Foundation Symposium 85, *Tinnitus,* Pitman, London, pp. 204–16

House, P.R. (1981b) 'Biofeedback Treatment of Tinnitus', *British Tinnitus Association Newsletter*, No. 12, iv–vi

House, P.R. (1981c) 'Personality of the Tinnitus Patient' in Ciba Foundation Symposium 85, *Tinnitus,* Pitman, London, pp. 193–203

House, W.F (1975) 'Menière's Disease: management and theory', *Otolaryngological Clinics of North America, 8,* 515–35

Hulshof, J.H. and Vermey, P. (1984) 'The Effects of Several Doses of Oral Tocainide hcl on Tinnitus: A Dose-finding Study', *Journal of Laryngology and Otology,* Supplement No. 9, Proceedings of the 2nd International Tinnitus Seminar, New York, 10 and 11 June, 1983, pp. 257–258

Jerger, J. (1970) 'Clinical experience with impedence audiometry', *Archives of Otolaryngology, 92,* 311–24

Johnson, R.M. and Mitchell, C.R. (1984) 'Tinnitus: Critical Bandwidth-masking Bands', *Journal of Laryngology and Otology,* Supplement No. 9, Proceedings of the 2nd International Tinnitus Seminar, New York, 10 and 11 June, 1983

Kemp, D. (1978) 'Stimulated acoustic emissions from within the human auditory system', *Journal of the Acoustical Society of America, 64,* 1386–91

Kemp, D. (1980) 'Ears Make Noises', *British Tinnitus Association Newsletter,* No. 5, iv

Kemp, D.T. (1981) 'Physiologically Active Cochlear Micromechanics — One Source of Tinnitus', in Ciba Foundation Symposium 85, *Tinnitus,* Pitman, London, pp. 54–76

Kennedy, P. (1984) 'British Tinnitus Association National Meeting of Self Help Groups', *British Tinnitus Association Newsletter,* No. 23, 4–5

Kim, D.O. and Molnar, C.E. (1979) 'A Population Study of Cochlear Nerve Fibres: Comparison of Spatial Distributions of Average-Rate and Phase Locking Measures of Responses to Single Tones', *Journal of Neurophysiology, 42,* 16–30

Kryter, K.D. (1970) *The effects of noise on man,* Academic Press, New York

Lackner, J.R. (1976) 'The Auditory Characteristics of Tinnitus Resulting from Cerebral Injury', *Experimental Neurology, 51,* 54–67

Lechtenberg, R. and Shulman, A. (1984) 'Benzodiazepines in the Treatment of Tinnitus', *The Journal of Laryngology and Otology,* Supplement No. 9, Proceedings of the 2nd International Tinnitus Seminar, New York, 10 and 11 June, 1983, pp. 271–76

Lesinski, S.G., Chambers, A.A., Komray, R., Keiser, M. and Khodadad, G. (1979) 'Why Not the Eighth Nerve? Neurovascular Compression — Probable Cause for Pulsatile Tinnitus', *Journal of Otolaryngology and Head and Neck Surgery, 87* (1), 89–94

Letowski, T.R. and Thompson, M.V. (1985) 'Interrupted Noise as a Tinnitus Masker: an annoyance study', *Ear and Hearing, 6* (2), 65–70

Liberman, M.C. and Kiang, N.Y.S. (1978) 'Acoustic Trauma in Cats', *Acta Otolaryngologica,* Supplement 358, pp. 1–63

Lind, M.G. and Lundquist, P.G. (1979), 'Tinnitus Caused by Bilateral Shunts from the Occipital Arteries to the Intracranial Veins — A Case Report', *Archives of Otorhinolaryngology, 222* (3), 229–34

Loavenbruck, A. (1980) 'Tinnitus Masking Devices: Safe and Effective?', *American Speech-Language-Hearing Association, 22* (10), 857–61

Longridge, N.S. (1979) 'A Tinnitus Clinic', *Journal of Otolaryngology, 8* (5), 390–5

Majumdar, B., Mason, S.M. and Gibbin, K.P. (1983) 'An Electrocochleographic Study of the Effects of Lignocaine on Patients with Tinnitus', *Clinical Otolaryngology, 8* (3), 175–80

Marchiando, A., Per-Lee, J.H. and Jackson, R.T. (1983) 'Tinnitus due to Idiopathic Stapedial Muscle Spasm', *Ear, Nose and Throat Journal, 62* (1), 8–13

Marks, N.J., Onisiphorou, C. and Trounce, J.R. (1981) 'The Effect of Single Doses of Amylobarbitone Sodium and Carbamazepine in Tinnitus', *Journal of Laryngology and Otology, 95* (9), 941–5

Martin, F.W. (1980) 'Intravenous Lignocaine Trials for Tinnitus Relief', *British Tinnitus Association Newsletter*, No. 8, i–iii

Martin, F.W. (1982) 'Adaptation of Drugs in the Management of Tinnitus', *British Tinnitus Association Newsletter*, No. 18, i–iii

Martin, F.W. and Colman, B.H. (1980) 'Tinnitus: A Double-blind Crossover Controlled Trial to Evaluate the Use of Lignocaine', *Clinical Otolaryngology, 5* (1), 3–11

Mayer, A.M., (1876) 'Research in Acoustics, *Philosophical Magazine, 11*, 500–7

Mathur, J.G. (1980) 'Hypothesis: Vascular Compression of the Cranial Nerve Roots (Letter)', *Medical Journal of Australia, 1* (8), 392

McCormick, M.S. and Thomas, J.N. (1981) 'Mexiletine in the Relief of Tinnitus: A Report on a Sequential Double-blind Crossover Trial', *Clinical Otolaryngology, 6* (4), 255–8

McFadden, D. (1982) *Tinnitus: Facts, Theories and Treatments*, National Academy Press, Washington, D.C.

McFadden, D. and Pasanen, E.G. (1980) 'Altered Psycho-physical Tuning Curves Following Exposure to a Noise Band with Steep Spectral Skirts', in G. van der Brink and F.A. Bilsen (eds.) *Psychophysical, Physiological, and Behavioural Studies in Hearing*, Delft University Press, Delft, the Netherlands

Meador, K.J., Stefadouros, M., Malik, A.J. and Swift, T.R. (1982) 'Self-heard Venous Bruit due to Increased Intercranial Pressure', *Lancet, 1* (8268), 391

Meikle, M. and Taylor-Walsh, E. (1984) 'Characteristics of Tinnitus and Related Observations in Over 1800 Tinnitus Clinical Patients', *Journal of Laryngology and Otology*, Supplement No. 9, Proceedings of the 2nd International Tinnitus Seminar, New York, 10 and 11 June, 1983, pp. 17–21

Melding, P.S. and Goodey, R.J. (1979) 'The Treatment of Tinnitus with Oral Anticonvulsants', *Journal of Laryngology and Otology, 93*, 111–22

Meyerhoff, W.L. and Shrewsbury, D. (1980) 'Rational Approaches to Tinnitus', *Geriatrics, 35* (10), 90–3

Miller, M.H. (1981) 'Tinnitus Amplification: The High Frequency Hearing

Aid', *Journal of Laryngology and Otology,* Supplement 4, 71–5

Miller, M.H. and Jakimetz, J.R. (1984) 'Noise Exposure, Hearing Loss, Speech Discrimination and Tinnitus', *Journal of Laryngology and Otology,* Supplement No. 9, Proceedings of the 2nd International Tinnitus Seminar, New York, 10 and 11 June, 1983, pp. 74–6

Moore, B.C.J. (1973) 'Frequency DLs for Short Duration Tones', *Journal of the Acoustical Society of America, 54,* 610–19

Mongan, E., Kelly, P., Nies, K., Porter, W.W. and Paulus, H.E. (1973) 'Tinnitus as an Indication of Therapeutic Serum Salicylate Levels', *Journal of the American Medical Association, 226* (2), 142–5

Nodar, R.H. (1972) 'Tinnitus Aurium in School Age Children: A Survey', *Auditory Research, 12,* 133

Nodar, R.H. and Le Zak, M.H.W. (1984) 'Paediatric Tinnitus (A Thesis Revisited)', *Journal of Laryngology and Otology,* Supplement No. 9, Proceedings of the 2nd International Tinnitus Seminar, New York, 10 and 11 June, 1983, pp. 234–5

Office of Population Censuses and Surveys (1980) *Classification of Occupations,* HMSO, London

Officer of Population Censuses and Surveys (1983) 'General Household Survey: The Prevalence of Tinnitus', OPCS, London

Patterson, R.D. (1976) 'Auditory Filter Shapes Derived with Noise Stimuli', *Journal of the Acoustic Society of America, 59,* 640–54

Penner, M.J. (1983) 'Variability in Matches to Subjective Tinnitus', *Journal of Speech and Hearing Research, 26* (2), 263–7

Portmann, M., Cazals, Y., Negrevergne, M. and Aran, J.M. (1979) 'Temporary Tinnitus Suppression in Man through Electrical Stimulation of the Cochlea', *Acta Otolaryngologica, 87* (3/4), 294–9

Pulec, J.L., Hodell, S.F. and Anthony, P.F. (1978) 'Tinnitus: Diagnosis and Treatment', *Annals of Otology, Rhinology and Laryngology, 87* (6 Pt. 1), 821–33

Robinson, M. (184) 'Tinnitus and Otosclerosis Surgery', *Journal of Laryngology and Otology,* Supplement No. 9, Proceedings of the 2nd International Tinnitus Seminar, New York, 10 and 11 June, 1983, pp. 294–8

Ronis, M.L. (1984) 'Alcohol and Dietary Influences on Tinnitus', *Journal of Laryngology and Otology,* Supplement No. 9, Proceedings of the 2nd International Tinnitus Seminar, New York, 10 and 11 June, 1983, pp. 242–6

Rubin, W. (1984) 'Tinnitus Evaluations: Aids to Daignosis and Treatment', *Journal of Laryngology and Otology,* Supplement No. 9, Proceedings of the 2nd International Tinnitus Seminar, New York, 10 and 11 June, 1983, pp. 178–80

Rutten, W.L.C. (1980) 'Evoked Acoustic Emissions from within Normal and Abnormal Human Ears: Comparison with Audiometric and Electrocochleographic Findings', *Hearing Research, 2,* 263–71

Schmiedt, R.A., Zwislocki, J.J. and Hamernik, R.. (1980) Effects of Hair Cell Lesions on Responses of Cochlear Nerve Fibres. I. Lesions, Tuning Curves, Two-tone Inhibition, and Responses to Trapezoidal-wave Patterns, *Journal of Neurophysiology, 43,* 16–30

Seebeck, A. (1841) 'Beobachtungen uber einige Bedingungen der Entstehung von Tonen', *Ann. Phys. Chem., 53,* 417–36

210

Scharf, B. (1970) 'Critical Bands', in J.V. Tobias (ed.) *Foundations of Modern Auditory Theory*, Academic, New York, Vol 1. Chapter 5, pp. 157–202

Schleuning, A. (1981) 'Neurotologic Evaluation of Subjective Idiopathic Tinnitus', *Journal of Laryngology and Otology*, Supplement 4, 99–101

Schouten, J.F. (1940) 'The Residue and the Mechanism of Hearing' *Prok, Kon. Nederl. Akad. Wetensch, 43*, 991–9

Schouten, J.F. (1970) 'The Residue Revisited' in R. Plomp and G.F. Smoorenburg (eds), *Frequency Analysis and Periodicity Detection in Hearing*, A.W. Sijthoff, Leiden

Shailer, M.J., Tyler, R.S. and Coles, R.R. (1981) 'Critical Masking Bands for Sensorineural Tinnitus', *Scandinavian Audiology, 10* (3), 157–62

Shea, J.J. (1981) 'Otosclerosis and Tinnitus', *Journal of Laryngology and Otology*, Supplement 4, 149–50

Shea, J.J. (1984) 'Medical Treatment of Tinnitus with Xylocaine^{TM} and Tocainide^{TM}', *Journal of Laryngology and Otology*, Supplement No. 9, Proceedings of the 2nd International Tinnitus Seminar, New York, 10 and 11 June, 1983, pp. 259–63

Shea, J.J. and Harell, M. (1978) 'Management of Tinnitus Aurium with Lidocaine and Carbamazepine', *Laryngoscope, 88* (9 Pt. 1), 1477–84

Shea, J.J., Emmett, J.R., Orchik, D.J., Mays, K. and Webb, W. (1981) 'Medical Treatment of Tinnitus', *Annals of Otology, Rhinology and Laryngology, 90* (6 Pt. 1), 601–9

Shucart, W.A. and Tenner, M. (1981) 'Tinnitus and Neurosurgical Disease', *Journal of Laryngology and Otology*, Supplement 4, 166–8

Shulman, A. (1981a) 'Subjective Idiopathic Tinnitus: A Review', *Journal of Laryngology and Otology*, Supplement 4, 1–9

Shulman, A. (1981) 'State of the Art: Identification and Treatment of Subjective Idiopathic Tinnitus', *Journal of Laryngology and Otology*, Supplement 4, 203–12

Shulman, A. (1984) 'Vestibular Test Battery Correlates and Tinnitus', *Journal of Laryngology and Otology*, Supplement No. 9, Proceedings of the 2nd International Tinnitus Seminar, New York, 10 and 11 June, 1983, pp. 181–3

Shulman, A. and Goldstein, B. (1984) 'Neurotologic Classification and Tinnitus', *Journal of Laryngology and Otology*, Supplement No. 9, Proceedings of the 2nd International Tinnitus Seminar, New York, 10 and 11 June, 1983, pp. 147–9

Shulman, A. and Seitz, M.R. (1981) 'Central Tinnitus — Diagnosis and Treatment, Observations Simultaneous Binaural Auditory Brain Responses with Monaural Stimulation in the Tinnitus Patient', *Laryngoscope, 91* (12), 2025–35

Shulman, A. *et al.* (1981) 'Panel Discussion: Acoustic Tumor and Tinnitus', *Journal of Laryngology and Otology*, Supplement 4, 143–8

Spitzer, J.B. (1981) 'Auditory Effects of Chronic Alcoholism', *Drug and Alcohol Dependence, 8* (4), 317–35

Stephens, S.D.G. (1984) 'The Treatment of Tinnitus — A Historical Perspective', *Journal of Laryngology and Otology, 98*, 963–72

Terry, A.M.P., Jones, D.M., Slater, R. and Davis, B.R. (1983) 'Parametric Studies of Tinnitus Masking and Residual Inhibition', *British Journal of Audiology, 17*, 245–56

Terry, A.M.P. and Jones, D.M. (1986) 'Preference for Potential Tinnitus Maskers: Results from Annoyance Ratings', *British Journal of Audiology*, 20, 277–97

Thomas, J.E. and Cody, D.T. (1981) 'Neurologic Perspectives of Otosclerosis', *Mayo Clinic Proceedings*, 56 (1), 17–18

Toland, A.D., Porubsky, E.S., Coker, N.J. and Adams, H.G. (1984) 'Velopharyngo-laryngeal Myoclonus: Evaluation of Objective Tinnitus and Extrathoracic Airway Obstruction', *Laryngoscope*, 94 (5 Pt. 1), 691–5

Turner, J.S. (1982) 'Treatment of Hearing Loss, Ear Pain and Tinnitus in Older Patients', *Geriatrics*, 37 (8), 107–11, 116, 118

Tyler, R.S. (1984) 'Does Tinnitus Originate from Hyperactive Nerve Fibres in the Cochlea?', *Journal of Laryngology and Otology*, Supplement No. 9, Proceedings of the 2nd International Tinnitus Seminar, New York, 10 and 11 June, 1983, pp. 38–44

Tyler, R.S. and Conrad-Armes, D. (1982) 'Spontaneous Acoustic Cochlear Emissions and Sensorineural Tinnitus', *British Journal of Audiology*, 16 (3), 193–4

Tyler, R.S. and Conrad-Armes, D. (1983) 'The Determination of Tinnitus Loudness Considering the Effects of Recruitment', *Journal of Speech and Hearing Research*, 26 (1), 59–72

Tyler, R.S. and Conrad-Armes, D. (1984) 'Masking of Tinnitus Compared to Masking of Pure Tones', *Journal of Speech and Hearing Research*, 27 (1), 106–11

Tyler, R.S., Babin, R.W. and Niebuhr, D.P. (1984) 'Some Observations on the Masking and Post-masking Effects of Tinnitus', *Journal of Laryngology and Otology*, Supplement No. 9, Proceedings of the 2nd International Tinnitus Seminar, New York, 10 and 11 June, 1983, pp. 150–6

Vernon, J. (1977) 'Attempts to Relieve Tinnitus', *Journal of the American Audiology Society*, 2 (4), 124–31

Vernon, J. (1978) 'The Other Noise Damage: Tinnitus', *Sound and Vibration*, 12 (5), 26

Vernon, J. (1979) 'What is Happening in U.S.A.', *British Tinnitus Association Newsletter*, No. 1, iv

Vernon, J. (1981) 'The History of Masking as Applied to Tinnitus', *Journal of Laryngology and Otology*, Supplement 4, 76–9

Vernon, J., Johnson, R. and Schleuning, A. (1980) 'The Characteristics and Natural History of Tinnitus in Menière's Disease', *Otolaryngologic Clinics of North America*, 13 (4), 611–19

Vernon, J. and Meikle, M.B. (1981) 'Tinnitus Masking: Unresolved Problems' in Ciba Foundation Symposium 85, *Tinnitus*, Pitman, London, pp. 239–62

Virtanen, H. (1983) 'Objective Tubal Tinnitus: A Report of Two Cases', *Journal of Laryngology and Otology*, 97 (9), 857–62

Walford, R.E. (1980) 'Research into Low Frequency Tinnitus', *British Tinnitus Association Newsletter*, No. 9, i–iv

Ward, W.D., Glorig, A. and Sklar, D.L. (1958) 'Dependence of Temporary Threshold Shift at Four Kc on Intensity and Time', *Journal of the Acoustical Society of America*, 30, 944–54

Wegel, R.L. and Lane, C.E. (1924) 'The Auditory Masking of One Pure Tone by Another and its Probable Relation to the Dynamics of the Inner

Ear, *Physical Review, 23,* series 2, 266–85

Whittaker, C.K. (1982) 'Letters To The Editor', *American Journal of Otology, 4* (2), 188

Whittaker, C.K. (1983) 'Letters To The Editor', *American Journal of Otology, 4* (3), 273

Williams, J.D. (1980) 'Unusual but Treatable Cause of Fluctuating Tinnitus', *Annals of Otology Rhinology and Laryngology, 89* (3 Pt. 1), 239–40

Wilson, J.P. (1980a) 'Model for Cochlear Echoes and Tinnitus Based on an Observed Electrical Correlate', *Hearing Research, 2* (2–4), 527–32

Wilson, J.P. (1980b) 'Evidence for a Cochlear Origin for Acoustic Re-emissions, Threshold Fine Structure and Tonal Tinnitus', *Hearing Research, 2* (3–4), 233–52

Wilson, J.P. and Sutton, G.J. (1981) 'Acoustic Correlates of Tonal Tinnitus' in Ciba Foundation Symposium 85, *Tinnitus,* Pitman, London, pp. 82–107

Wood, K.A., Webb, W.L., Orchik, D.J. and Shea, J.J. (1983) 'Intractable Tinnitus: Psychiatric Aspects of Treatment', *Psychosomatics, 24* (6), 559–65

Ylikoski, J. (1979) 'Morphological Findings in Eight Nerve and Vestibular Organs', *Journal of Oto-Rhino-Laryngology, 41,* 26–32

Young, I.M. and Lowry, L.D. (1983) 'Incurrence and Alterations in Contralateral Tinnitus Following Monaural Exposure to a Pure Tone', *Journal of the Acoustical Society of America, 73* (6), 2219–21

Zurek, P.M. (1981) 'Spontaneous narrowband acoustic signals emitted by the human ears', *Journal of the Acoustical Society of America, 69,* 514–23

213

Bibliography of Additional Items on Tinnitus

Ahmad, R., Raichura, N., Kilbane, V. and Whitfield, E. (1982) 'Vancomycin: a Reappraisal — Letter to the Editor', *British Medical Journal, 284* (6333), 1953-4

Ambrosino, S.V. (1981) 'Neuropsychiatric Aspects of Tinnitus', *Journal of Laryngology and Otology,* Supplement 4, 169-72

Anderson, B. (1981) 'I Suddenly Realised That I Had These Noises', *British Tinnitus Association Newsletter,* No. 14, i–ii

Andreasson, L., Harris, S. and Ivarsson, A. (1978) 'Pulse Volume Recordings in Outer Ear Canal in Pulse Synchronous Tinnitus. A Comparison Between Ears with Glomus Tumour, Serious Otitis Media, and Normal Ears', *Acta Otolaryngologica, 86* (3–4), 241–7

Anon (1979) 'Treatment of Tinnitus', *British Medical Journal, 1* (6176), 1445–6

Anon (1980) 'Editorial: the Treatment of Tinnitus', *Clinical Otolaryngology, 5* (1), 1–2

Anon (1984) 'Tinnitus (Editorial)', *Lancet, 1* (8376), 543–5

Aran, J.M. (1981) 'Electrical Stimulation of the Auditory System and Tinnitus Control', *Journal of Laryngology and Otology,* Supplement 4, 153–61

Aran, J.M., Sauvage, R.C. de and Erre, J.P. (1984) 'Perspectives in Electrical Stimulation of the Ear (Experimental Studies)', *Journal of Laryngology and Otology,* Supplement No. 9, Proceedings of the 2nd International Tinnitus Seminar, New York, 10 and 11 June, 1983, pp. 132–6

Arenberg, L.K. and Balkany, T.J. (1984) 'Objective Pulsatile Tinnitus: Vascular Basis', *Journal of Laryngology and Otology,* Supplement No. 9, Proceedings of the 2nd International Tinnitus Seminar, New York, 10 and 11 June, 1983, pp. 84–93

Arenberg, L.K., Gibson, S.A., Van de Water, S.M. and Balkany, T.J. (1984) 'The Effect of Endolymphatic System Surgery on Tinnitus in Menière's Disease and Hydrops', *Journal of Laryngology and Otology,* Supplement No. 9, Proceedings of the 2nd International Tinnitus Seminar, New York, 10 and 11 June, 1983, pp. 229–310

Atherley, G.R.C., Hempstock, T.I. and Noble, W.G. (1968) 'Study of Tinnitus Induced Temporarily by Noise', *Journal of the Acoustical Society of America, 44,* 1503–6

Bailey, Q. (1979) 'Audiological Aspects of Tinnitus', *Australian Journal of Audiology, 1,* 19–23

Ballantyne, J. and Groves, J. (1972) *Scott-Brown's Diseases of the Ear, Nose and Throat* (3rd Edn), Butterworth, London

Ballantyne, J.C. (1977) 'The Hearing Ear: Variations on a Theme of Helmholtz', *Proceedings of the Royal Society of Medicine, 70,* 128–38

Bender, D.R. and Mueller, H.G. (1981) 'Military Noise Inducing Hearing Loss: Incidence and Managements', *Military Medicine, 146,* 434–7

Berlin, C.I. and Shearer, P.D. (1981) 'Electrophysiological Simulation of

Tinnitus' in Ciba Foundation Symposium 85, *Tinnitus*, Pitman, London, pp. 139–50

Blanchard, E.B., Young, L.D. and Jackson, M.S. (1974) 'Clinical Applications of Biofeedback Training: A Review of Evidence', *Archives of General Psychiatry, 30*, 573–89

Blayney, A.W., Phillips, M.S., Guy, A.M. and Colman, B.H. (1985) 'A Sequential Double Blind Cross-over Trial of Tocainide Hydrochloride in Tinnitus', *Clinical Otolaryngology, 10* (2), 97–101

Borton, T.E., Moore, W.H. Jr. and Clark, S.R. (1981) 'Electromyographic Feedback Treatment for Tinnitus Aurium', *Journal of Speech and Hearing Disorders, 46* (1), 39–45

Brackmann, D.E. (1981) 'Reduction of Tinnitus in Cochlea-implant Patients', *Journal of Laryngology and Otology*, Supplement No. 4, 163–5

British Tinnitus Association (1981) 'Maskers on the National Health Service', *British Tinnitus Association Newsletter*, No. 13, i–iii

British Tinnitus Association (1983) 'A Signpost to the Future', *British Tinnitus Association Newsletter*, No. 19, i *et seq.*

Buckwalter, J.A., Sasaki, C.T., Virapongse, C., Kier, E.L. and Bauman, N. (1983) 'Pulsatile Tinnitus Arising from Jugular Megabulb Deformity: a Treatment Rationale', *Laryngoscope, 93*, 1534–9

Budzynski, T., Stoyva, J. and Adler, C. (1980) 'Feedback-induced Muscle Relaxation: Application to Tension Headache', *Journal of Behaviour Therapy and Experimental Psychiatry, 1*, 205–11

Bunch, C.C. (1937) 'Nerve Deafness of Known Pathology or Aetiology: the Diagnosis of Occupational or Traumatic Deafness, a Historical and Audiometric Study', *Laryngoscope, 47*, 615–91

Burns, E.M. (1984) 'A Comparison of Variability Among Measurements of Subjective Tinnitus and Objective Stimuli', *Audiology, 23* (4), 426–40

Cahani, M., Paul, G. and Shahar, A. (1983) 'Tinnitus Pitch and Acoustic Trauma', *Audiology, 22* (4), 357–63

Cahani, M., Paul, G. and Shahar, A. (1984) 'Tinnitus Asymmetry', *Audiology, 23* (1), 127–35

Carbary, L.J. (1980) 'Tuning Out Tinnitus', *Journal of Nursing Care, 13* (8), 8–11

Carmen, R. and Svihovec, D. (1984) 'Relaxation-biofeedback in the Treatment of Tinnitus', *American Journal of Otology, 5* (5), 376–81

Caro, A.Z. (1975) 'Dimethyl Sulfoxide Therapy in Subjective Tinnitus of Unknown Origin', *Annals of the New York Academy of Sciences', 243*, 468–74

Cazals, Y., Negrevergne, M. and Aran, J.M. (1978) 'Electrical Stimulation of the Cochlea in Man: Hearing Induction and Tinnitus Suppression', *Journal of the American Audiology Society, 3* (5), 209–13

Charles, W.J. (1977) 'Electroconvulsive Therapy (Letter)', *British Journal of Psychiatry, 131*, 551

Chouard, C.H., Mayer, B. and Maridat, D. (1981) 'Transcutaneous Electrotherapy for Severe Tinnitus', *Acta Otolaryngologica, 91* (5/6), 415–22

Chung, D.Y., Gannan, R.P. and Mason, K. (1984) 'Factors Affecting the Prevalence of Tinnitus', *Audiology, 23*, 441–52

215

Clark, S.R. and Smith, C.R. (1981) 'Industrial Tinnitus', *Hearing Aid Journal*, *34*, 36–7

Claussen, C.F. and Claussen, E. (1984) 'Objective Neural-otological Investigations in Patients with Vertigo and Tinnitus Using ENG and Acoustically Evoked Responses', *Archives of Oto-Rhino-Laryngology*, *239*, 101

Clemis, J.D. (1984) 'Tinnitus and Impedance Audiometry', *Journal of Laryngology and Otology*, Supplement No. 9, Proceedings of the 2nd International Tinnitus Seminar, New York, 10 and 11 June, 1983, pp. 161–4

Coates, A. (1982) 'Learning to Cope', *British Tinnitus Association Newsletter*, No. 16, iii–iv

Cochran, J.H., Jr., Kosmicki, P.W. and Colarado, D. (1979) 'Tinnitus as a Presenting Symptom in Pernicious Anaemia', *Annals of Otology Rhinology and Laryngology*, *88* (2 Pt. 1), 297

Cole, F. (1978) 'A Curious Case of Tinnitus', *Nebraska Medical Journal*, *64* (2), 33

Coles, R.R.A. (1982) 'Noise-induced Tinnitus', *Proceedings of the Institute of Acoustics*, *64*, 1–5

Coles, R.R.A., Baskill, J.L. and Sheldrake, J.B. (1985) 'Measurement and Management of Tinnitus. Part II. Management', *Journal of Laryngology and Otology*, *99* (1), 1–10

Coles, R.R.A. and Hoare, N.W. (1985) 'Noise-induced Hearing Loss and the Dentist', *British Dental Journal*, *159* (7), 209–18

Collins, E.G. (1944) 'Injury to the Ears Among Battle Casualties of the Western Desert', *Journal of Laryngology and Otology*, *59*, 1015

Collins, E.G. (1948) 'Aural Trauma Caused by Gunfire', *Journal of Laryngology and Otology*, *63*, 358–90

Davis, A.C. (1983) 'Hearing Disorders in the Population: First Phase Findings of the MRC National Study of Hearing', In M.E. Lutman and M. Haggard (eds.), *Hearing Science and Hearing Disorders*, Academic Press, New York, pp. 35–60

Dawes, J.D.K. (1984) 'What Treatment is Advised for a 70 Year Old Patient With Severe Bilateral Tinnitus Uncontrolled by Prochlorperazine or Trifluoperazine?' (Any Questions), *British Medical Journal*, *289*, (6436), 42

Decker, T.N. and Fritsch, J.H. (1982) 'Objective Tinnitus in the Dog', *Journal of the American Veterinary Medical Association*, *180* (1), 74

DeWeese, D. and Vernon, J. (1975) 'Hearing Instruments', *American Tinnitus Association*, *26* (12), 38–40

Dickter, A.E., Durrant, J.D. and Ronis, M.L. (1981) 'Correlation of the Complaint of Tinnitus with Central Auditory Testing', *Journal of Laryngology and Otology*, Supplement No. 4, 52–9

Dornan, J.D. (1984) 'Some Hazards Associated with Spring Correction', *Journal of the Society of Occupational Medicine*, *34* (1), 33–4

Douek, E. (1981) 'Conclusion', *Journal of Laryngology and Otology*, Supplement No. 4, pp. 213–16

Douek, E. (1981) 'Cochleo-vestibular Correlates of Tinnitus: Tinnitogram', *Journal of Laryngology and Otology*, Supplement No. 4, 107–10

Douek, E. (1984) 'Loudness Intensity and Tinnitus Frequency', *Journal of*

Laryngology and Otology, Supplement No. 9, Proceedings of the 2nd International Tinnitus Seminar, New York, 10 and 11 June, 1983, pp. 67–8

Douek, E. (1984) 'Electrical Stimulation of the Inner Ear — Auditory Tinnitus Suppression and Speech Discrimination', *Journal of Laryngology and Otology,* Supplement No. 9, Proceedings of the 2nd International Tinnitus Seminar, New York, 10 and 11 June, 1983, pp. 137–8

Douek, E. (1984) 'Conclusion', *Journal of Laryngology and Otology,* Supplement No. 9, Proceedings of the 2nd International Tinnitus Seminar, New York, 10 and 11 June, 1983, pp. 321–2

Drake, T.E. (1974) 'Letter: Reaction to Gentamicin Sulfate Cream', *Archives of Dermatology, 110* (4), 638

Duckert, L.G. and Rees, T.S. (1983) 'Treatment of Tinnitus with Intravenous Lidocaine: a Double-blind Randomized Trial', *Otolaryngology and Head and Neck Surgery, 91,* 550–5

Duckert, L.G. and Rees, T.S. (1984) 'Placebo Effect in Tinnitus Management', *Otolaryngology and Head and Neck Surgery, 92* (6), 697–9

Duckro, P.N., Pollard, C.A., Bray, H.D. and Scheiter, L. (1984) 'Comprehensive Behavioral Management of Complex Tinnitus: a Case Illustration', *Biofeedback and Self Regulation, 9* (4) 459–69

Durrant, J.D. (1981) 'Auditory Physiology and an Auditory Physiologist's View of Tinnitus', *Journal of Laryngology and Otology,* Supplement No. 4, pp. 21–8

Ellis, P.D.M. and Wright, J.L.W. (1974) 'Acoustic Neuroma: A Plea for Early Diagnosis and Treatment', *Journal of Laryngology and Otology, 88,* 1095

Emmett, J.R. and Shea, J.J. (1980) 'Treatment of Tinnitus with Tocainide Hydrochloride', *Otolaryngology and Head and Neck Surgery, 88,* 442–6

Emmett, J.R. and Shea, J.J. (1984) 'Medical Treatment of Tinnitus', *Journal of Laryngology and Otology,* Supplement No. 9, Proceedings of the 2nd International Tinnitus Seminar, New York, 10 and 11 June, 1983, pp. 264–70

Elner, A., Ingelstedt, S. and Ivarsson (1971) 'The Elastic Properties of the Tympanic Membrane System', *Acta Otolaryngologica, 72,* 397–403

Englesson, S., Larsson, B., Lindquist, N.G., Lyttkens, L. and Stahle, J. (1976) 'Accumulation of 14C-Lidocaine in the Inner Ear. Preliminary Clinical Experience Utilizing Intravenous Lidocaine in the Treatment of Severe Tinnitus', *Acta Otolaryngologica, 82* (3–4), 297–300

Epley, J.M. (1981) 'Electronic Probe for Eustachian Tube Patency and Objective Tinnitus, *Otolaryngology and Head and Neck Surgery, 89* (5), 854–5

Evans, D.L. and Golden, R.N. (1981) 'Protriptyline and Tinnitus', *Journal of Clinical Psychopharmacology, 1* (6), 404–6

Feldmann, H. (1981) 'Homolateral and Contralateral Masking of Tinnitus', *Journal of Laryngology and Otology,* Supplement No. 4, pp. 60–70

Feldmann, H. (1984) 'Suppression of Tinnitus by Electrical Stimulation: A Contribution to the History of Medicine', *Journal of Laryngology and Otology,* Supplement No. 9, Proceedings of the 2nd International Tinnitus Seminar, New York, 10 and 11 June, 1983, pp. 123–4

Feldmann, H. (1984) 'Tinnitus Masking Curves (Updates and Review),

Journal of Laryngology and Otology, Supplement No. 9, Proceedings of the 2nd International Tinnitus Seminar, New York, 10 and 11 June, 1983, pp. 157–60

Formby, C. and Gjerdingen, D.B. (1980) 'Pure-tone Masking of Tinnitus', *Audiology, 19* (6), 519–35

Fowler, E.P. (1939) 'The Use of Threshold & Louder Sounds in Clinical Diagnosis and the Prescribing of Hearing Aids. New Methods for Accurately Determining the Threshold for Bone Conduction and for Measuring Tinnitus and its Effects on Obstructive and Neural Deafness', *Laryngoscope, 48,* 572–88

Fowler, E.P. (1944) 'Head Noises in Normal and in Disordered Ears', *American Laryngological, Rhinological and Otological Society, 39,* 498–503

Fox, M.S. and Bunn, J.H. (1979) 'Workers' Compensation Aspects of Noise Induced Hearing Loss', *Otolaryngologic Clinics of North America, 12,* 705–24

Gejrot, T. (1963) 'Intravenous Xylocaine in the Treatment of Attacks of Menière's Disease', *Acta Otolaryngologica,* Supplement No. 118, 190–5

Gerber, K.E., Nehemkis, A.M., Charter, R.A. and Jones H.C. (1985) 'Is Tinnitus a Psychological Disorder?' *International Journal of Psychiatry in Medicine, 15* (1), 81–7

Ghose, P. and Sardana, D.S. (1970) 'Tinnitogram and its Localising Value', *Indian Journal of Otolaryngology, 22,* 24–30

Gibson, R. (1973) 'Tinnitus in Paget's Disease with External Carotid Ligation', *Journal of Laryngology and Otology, 87* (3), 299–301

Goldstein, B. and Shulman, A. (1981) 'Tinnitus Classification: Medical Audiologic Assessment', *Journal of Laryngology and Otology,* Supplement No. 4, 33–8

Goodhill, V. (1954) 'Otology Aspects', *Transactions of American Academy of Ophthalmology and Otolaryngology, 58,* 529–32

Goodwin, P.E. and Johnson, R.M. (1980) 'A Comparison of Reaction Times to Tinnitus and Nontinnitus Frequencies', *Ear and Hearing, 1* (3), 148–55

Graham, J.M. (1981) 'Tinnitus in Children with Hearing Loss', in Ciba Foundation Symposium 85, *Tinnitus,* Pitman, London, pp. 172–92

Graham, J.M. (1981) 'Tinnitus and Deafness of Sudden Onset: Electrocochleographic Findings in 100 Patients', *Journal of Laryngology and Otology,* Supplement No. 4, 111–16

Graham, J.M. and Butler, J. (1984) 'Tinnitus in Children', *Journal of Laryngology and Otology.* Supplement No. 9, Proceedings of the 2nd International Tinnitus Seminar, New York, 10 and 11 June, 1983, pp. 235–41

Graham, M.D., Sataloff, R.T. and Kemink, J.L. (1984) 'Tinnitus in Menière's Disease: Response Titration to Streptomycin Therapy', *Journal of Laryngology and Otology,* Supplement No. 9, Proceedings of the 2nd International Tinnitus Seminar, New York, 10 and 11 June, 1983, pp. 281–6

Grossan, M. (1976) 'Treatment of Subjective Tinnitus with Biofeedback', *Ear, Nose and Throat Journal, 55* (10), 314–18

Gullikson, J.S. (1978) 'Tinnitus and the Dentist', *Journal of Orgon Dental Association, 47* (4), 8–9

Gulya, A.J. and Suknecht, H.F. (1984) 'A Large Artery in the Apical Region of the Cochlea of a Man with Pulsatile Tinnitus', [Letter], *American Journal of Otology, 5* (3), 262

Hallam, R. (1985) 'Tinnitus Research at the Audiology Centre, Royal National Throat, Nose and Ear Hospital', *Soundbarrier*, No. 5, British Tinnitus Association Newsletter, No. 29, 18

Hallam, R.S. and Jakes, S.C. (1985) 'Tinnitus: Differential Effects of Therapy in a Single Case', *Behaviour Research and Therapy, 23* (6), 691–4

Hallam, R.S. and Stephens, S.D. (1985) 'Vestibular Disorder and Emotional Distress', *Journal of Psychosomatic Research, 29* (4), 407–13

Hallam, R.S., Jakes, S.C., Chambers, C. and Hinchcliffe, R. (1985) 'A Comparison of Different Methods for Assessing the "Intensity" of Tinnitus', *Acta Otolaryngologica, 99* (5–6), 501–8

Hamberger, C.A. and Liden, C.A. (1951) 'The Prognosis in Hearing Injuries Following Acoustic Shot Traumata', *Acta Otolaryngologica, 39,* 160–5

Hanson, D.G. and Paparella, M.M. (1975) 'Metabolic Hearing Disorders — The Medical Treatment of Deafness', *Nervous System, 3,* 253–62

Harris, S. Brismar, J. and Cronqvist, S. (1979) 'Pulsatile Tinnitus and Therapeutic Embolization', *Acta Otolaryngologica, 88* (3–4), 220–6

Hatton, D.S., Erulkar, S.D. and Rosenberg, P.E. (1960) 'Some Preliminary Observations on the Effect of Galvanic Current on Tinnitus Aurium', *Laryngoscope, 70,* 123–30

Hazell, J.W.P. (1979) 'First International Tinnitus Seminar', *British Tinnitus Association Newsletter,* No. 2, iii–vi

Hazell, J.W.P. (1980) 'Tinnitus Research in the USA', *British Tinnitus Association Newsletter,* No. 4, iii–vii

Hazell, J.W.P. (1981) 'Medical Research', *British Tinnitus Association Newsletter,* No. 12, ii–iii

Hazell, J.W.P. (1981) 'A Tinnitus Synthesizer: Physiological Considerations', *Journal of Laryngology and Otology,* Supplement No. 4, 187–95

Hazell, J.W.P. (1983) 'Tinnitus', *Modern Medicine, 28,* 9–10

Hazell, J.W.P. (1983) 'Tinnitus', *Medicine International, 1,* 1342–3

Hazell, J.W.P. (1983) 'The General Household Survey of Tinnitus', *British Tinnitus Association Newsletter,* No. 20, vii–viii

Hazell, J.W.P. (1984) 'Spontaneous Cochlear Acoustic Emissions and Tinnitus: Clinical Experience in the Tinnitus Patient', *Journal of Laryngology and Otology,* Supplement No. 9, Proceedings of the 2nd International Tinnitus Seminar, New York, 10 and 11 June, 1983, pp. 106–10

Hazell, J.W.P. (1986) 'Management of Tinnitus: Discussion Paper', *Journal of the Royal Society of Medicine, 78* (1), 56–60

Hazell, J.W.P., Graham, J.M. and Rothera, M.P. (1985) 'Electrical Stimulation of the Cochlea and Tinnitus' in R.A. Schindler and M.M. Merzenich (eds.), *Cochlear Implants: Current Status and Future*, Raven Press, New York

Hazell, J.W.P., Williams, G.R. and Sheldrake, J.B. (1981) 'Tinnitus Maskers — Successes and Failures: a Report on the State of the Art', *Journal of Laryngology and Otology*, Supplement No. 4, 80–7

Hicks, K.W. (1978) 'Gnathology and Tinnitus' (Letter), *Journal of the American Medical Association, 239* (9), 830

Hinchcliffe, R. and Chambers, C. (1983) 'Loudness of Tinnitus: an Approach to Measurement', *Advances in Otorhinolaryngology, 29,* 163–73

Hochberg, I. and Waltzman, S. (1972) 'Comparison of Pulsed and Continuous Tone Thresholds in Patients with Tinnitus', *Audiology, 11* (5), 337–42

Holgate, R.C., Wortzman, G., Noyek, A.M., Makerewicz, L. and Coates, R.M. (1977) 'Pulsatile Tinnitus: The Role of Angiography', *Journal of Otolaryngology (Suppl), 6* (3), 49–62

House, J.W. (1978) 'Treatment of Severe Tinnitus with Biofeedback Training', *Laryngoscope, 88* (3), 406–12

House, J.W. (1984) 'Effects of Electrical Stimulation on Tinnitus', *Journal of Laryngology and Otology*, Supplement No. 9, Proceedings of the 2nd International Tinnitus Seminar, New York, 10 and 11 June, 1983, pp. 139–40

House, J.W., Miller, L. and House, P.R. (1977) 'Severe Tinnitus: Treatment with Biofeedback Training (Results in 41 Cases)', *Transactions of the American Academy of Opthalmology and Otolaryngology, 84* (4, Pt. 1), 697–703

House, P.R. (1984) 'Personality of the Tinnitus Patient', *Journal of Laryngology and Otology*, Supplement No. 9, Proceedings of the 2nd International Tinnitus Seminar, New York, 10 and 11 June, 1983, pp. 233

Huizing, E.H. and Spoor, A. (1973) 'An Unusual Type of Tinnitus. Production of a High Tone by the Ear', *Archives of Otolaryngology, 98* (2), 134–6

Hulshof, J.H. (1983) 'Drug Therapy of Tinnitus: The Effect of Intravenous Lignocaine and Oral Tocainide on Tinnitus' (Abstract), *Clinical Otolaryngology, 8,* 433

Hulshof, J.H. and Vermeij, P. (1985) 'The Value of Carbamazepine in the Treatment of Tinnitus', *Journal of Oto-Rhino-Laryngology and its Related Specialities, 47* (5), 262–6

Hvidegaard, T. and Brask, T. (1984) 'Objective Venous Tinnitus. A Case Report', *Journal of Laryngology and Otology, 98* (2), 189–91

Ince, L.P., Greene, R.Y., Alba, A. and Zaretsky, H.H. (1984) 'Learned Self-control of Tinnitus through a Matching-to-Sample Feedback Technique: a Clinical Investigation', *Journal of Behavioral Medicine, 7* (4), 355–65

Ireland, C.E., Wilson, P.H., Tonkin, J.P. and Platt-Hepworth, S. (1985) 'Evaluation of Relaxation Training in the Treatment of Tinnitus', *Behaviour Research and Therapy, 23* (4), 423–30

Israel, J.M., Connelly, J.S., McTigue, S.T., Brummett, R.E. and Brown, J. (1982) 'Lidocaine in the Treatment of Tinnitus Aurium. A Double-blind Study', *Archives of Otolaryngology, 108* (8), 471–3

Jackson, P. (1983) 'Tinnitus in the Elderly', in R. Hinchcliffe (ed.),

Hearing and Balance in the Elderly, Churchill Livingstone, Edinburgh, pp. 159–73

Jakes, S.C., Hallam, R.S., Chambers, C. and Hinchcliffe, R. (1985), 'A Factor Analytical Study of Tinnitus Complaint Behaviour', *Audiology*, 24 (3), 195–206

Jakes, S.C., Hallam, R.S., Chambers, C.C. and Hinchcliffe, R. (1986) 'Matched and Self-reported Loudness of Tinnitus: Methods and Sources of Er' *Audiology*, 25 (2), 92–100

Johnson, R.M. and Goodwin, P. (1981) 'The Use of Audiometric Tests in the Management of the Tinnitus Patient', *Journal of Laryngology and Otology*, Supplement No. 4, 48–51

Kauer, J.S., Nemitz, J.W. and Sasaki, C.T. (1982) 'Tinnitus Aurium: Fact . . . or Fancy', *Laryngoscope*, 92 (12), 1401–7

Keller, A.P. Jr. (1974) 'An Oscillographic Study of an Objective Tinnitus', *Laryngoscope*, 84 (6), 998–1003

Kemp, S. and Plaisted, I.D. (1986) 'Tinnitus Induced by Tones', *Journal of Speech and Hearing Research*, 29 (1), 65–70

Kennedy, P. (1982) 'Group Representatives Meet in London', *British Tinnitus Association Newsletter*, No. 17, vi

Kimura, Y. (1984) 'Tinnitus Without Hearing Loss', *Otolaryngology*, 47, 819–25

King, D.C. (1981) 'But What Do Maskers Actually Do?', *British Tinnitus Association Newsletter*, No. 13, iii–iv

Kirtley, P. (1980) 'Relaxation', *British Tinnitus Association Newsletter*, No. 9, viii–ix

Kudo, T. and Ito, K. (1984) 'Microvascular Decompression of the Eighth Cranial Nerve for Disabling Tinnitus Without Vertigo: A Case Report', *Neurosurgery*, 14 (3), 338–40

Lamprecht, J. and Morgenstern, C. (1984) 'A Simple Method for the Differentiation of Tonal Tinnitus', *Archives of Oto-Rhino-Laryngology*, 239, 120

Lancet (1984) 'Tinnitus' [Editorial], *Lancet*, 1 (8376), 543–5

Larsson, B., Lyttkens, L. and Waterstrom, S.A. (1984) 'Tocainide and Tinnitus. Clinical Effect and Site of Action', *Journal of Oto-Rhino-Laryngology and Related Specialities*, 46 (1), 24–33

Laudadio, P., Rinaldi, A., Ceroni, R. and Cerasoli, P.T. (1984) 'Metastatic Malignant Melanoma in the Parotid Gland', *Journal of Oto-Rhino-Laryngology and Related Specialities*, 46, 42–9

Lauten, G.J. and Neal, T.F. (1978) 'Enlarged Internal Auditory Canals: Case Report and Review', *Ear, Nose and Throat Journal*, 57 (12), 50–5

Lechtenberg, R. and Shulman, A. (1984) 'The Neurologic Implications of Tinnitus', *Archives of Neurology*, 41 (7), 718–21

Leveque, H. Bialostozky, F., Blanchard, C.L. and Suter, C.M. (1979) 'Tympanometry in the Evaluation of Vascular Lesions of the Middle Ear and Tinnitus of Vascular Origin', *Laryngoscope*, 89 (8), 1197–218

Levitt, H. (1984) 'Models of the Auditory System and Tinnitus', *Journal of Laryngology and Otology*, Supplement No. 9, Proceedings of the 2nd International Tinnitus Seminar, New York, 10 and 11 June, 1983, pp. 25–30

Lindberg, P., Lyttkens, L., Melin, L. and Scott, B. (1984) 'Tinnitus —

Incidence and Handicap', *Scandinavian Audiology, 13* (4), 287–91

Linday, M. (1983) 'The Roaring Deafness', *Nursing Times, 79* (5), 61–3

Linquist, N.L. (1973) 'Accumulation of Drugs on Melanin', *Acta Radiologica,* Supplement No. 325, 78–83

Litman, R.S. and Hausman, S.A. (1982) 'Bilateral Palatal Myoclonus', *Laryngoscope, 92* (10), 1187–9

Loeb, M. and Smith, R.P. (1967) 'Relation of Induced Tinnitus to Physical Characteristics of the Inducing Stimuli', *Journal of the Acoustical Society of America, 42,* 453–5

Lyons, G.D., Melancon, B.B., Kearby, N.L. and Zimny, M. (1976) 'The Otological Aspects of Palatal Myoclonus', *Laryngoscope, 86* (7), 930–6

Lyttkens, L., Larsson, B. and Wasterstrom, S.A. (1984) 'Local Anaesthetics and Tinnitus. Proposed Peripheral Mechanisms of Action of Lidocaine', *Journal of Oto-Rhino-Laryngology and Related Specialities, 46* (1), 17–23

Macleod-Morgan, C., Court, J. and Roberts, R. (1982) 'Cognitive Restructuring: A Technique for the Relief of Chronic Tinnitus', *Australian Journal of Clinical and Experimental Hypnosis, 10,* 27–33

Maddox, H.E. 3rd and Porter, T.H. (1981) 'Evaluation of the Tinnitus Masker', *American Journal of Otology, 2* (3), 199–203

Man, A. and Naggan, L. (1981) 'Characteristics of Tinnitus in Acoustic Trauma', *Audiology, 20* (1), 72–8

Marco, L.A. (1978) 'Narcolepsy with Tinnitus Aura: Interpretation', *International Journal of Psychiatry and Medicine, 9* (3–4), 275–80

Marks, N.J., Karl, H. and Onisiphorou, C. (1985) 'A Controlled Trial of Hypnotherapy in Tinnitus', *Clinical Otolaryngology, 10* (1), 43–6

Marlowe, F.I. (1973) 'Effective Treatment of Tinnitus through Hypnotherapy', *American Journal of Clinical Hypnosis, 15* (3), 162–5

Marsh, M.N., Holbrook, I.B., Clark, C. and Shaffer, J.L. (1981) 'Tinnitus in a Patient with Beta-thalassaemia Intermedia on Long-term Treatment with Desferrioxamine', *Postgraduate Medical Journal, 57* (671), 582–4

Martin, M.C. (1980) 'Tinnitus Maskers', *British Tinnitus Association Newsletter,* No. 6, i–vi

Martin, M.C. (1981) 'BTA Tinnitus Meeting', *British Tinnitus Association Newsletter,* No. 11, i–iii

Matz, G.J. (1975) 'Toxic Cochlear and Vestibular Disorders', *Nervous System, 3,* 333–49

Meador, K.M. and Swift, T.R. (1984) 'Tinnitus from Intracranial Hypertension', *Neurology, 34,* 1258–61

Meikle, M. and Whitney, S. (1984) 'Computer-assisted Analysis of Reported Tinnitus Sounds', *Journal of Laryngology and Otology,* Supplement No. 9, Proceedings of the 2nd International Tinnitus Seminar, New York, 10 and 11 June, 1983, pp. 188–92

Melding, P.S., Goodey, R.J. and Thorne, P.R. (1978) 'The Use of Intravenous Lignocaine in the Diagnosis and Treatment of Tinnitus', *Journal of Laryngology and Otology, 92* (2), 115–21

Merluzzi, F. (1983) 'Occupational Deafness' in L. Parmeggiani (ed.) *Encyclopaedia of Occupational Health and Safety,* Vol. 1, International Labour Office, Geneva, pp. 593–6

Mesolella, C., D'Errico, G., Barillari, U. and Testa, B. (1984) 'Objective

Tinnitus Due to Peritubal Myoclonus. A Case Report', *Journal of Oto-Rhino-Laryngology and Related Specialities, 46* (1), 50–6

Michel, R.G., Drawbaugh, E.J and Thaddeus, H.P. (1976) 'A Practical Approach to the Treatment of Subjective Tinnitus', *Otolaryngology, 55* (3), 48–51

Michelson, R.P., Merzenich, M.M., Schindler, R.A. and Schindler, D.N. (1975) 'Present Status and Future Development of the Cochlear Prosthesis', *Annals of Otology, Rhinology, and Laryngology, 84,* 494–8

Miles, S.W. (1980) 'Amitriptyline Side Effect (Letter)', *New Zealand Medical Journal, 92* (664), 66–7

Miller, S.M. (1982) 'Erythromycin Ototoxicity', *Medical Journal of Australia, 2* (5), 242–3

Mills, R.P. and Cherry, J.R. (1984) 'Subjective Tinnitus in Children with Otological Disorders', *International Journal of Paediatric Otorhinolaryngology, 7* (1), 21–7

Mitchell, C. (1983) 'The Masking of Tinnitus with Pure Tones', *Audiology, 22* (1), 73–87

Mitchell, C., Brummett, R., Himes, D. and Vernon, J. (1973) 'Electro-physiological Study of the Effect of Sodium Salicylate Upon the Cochlea', *Archives in Otolaryngology, 98,* 197–301

Mitchell, P.L., Moffat, D.A. and Fallside, F. (1984) 'Computer-aided Tinnitus Characterization', *Clinical Otolaryngology, 9* (1), 35–42

Moller, A.R. (1984) 'Pathophysiology of Tinnitus', *Annals of Otology Rhinology and Laryngology, 93* (1, Pt. 1), 39–44

Moller, P., Grevstad, A.O. and Kristoffersen, T. (1976) 'Ultrasonic Scaling of Maxillary Teeth Causing Tinnitus and Temporary Hearing Shifts', *Journal of Clinical Periodontology, 3* (2), 123–7

Moore, B.C.J. (1982) *An Introduction to the Psychology of Hearing,* Academic Press, New York

Moroso, M.J. and Blair, R.L. (1983) 'A Review of Cis-platinum Ototoxicity', *Journal of Otolaryngology, 12* (6), 365–9

Murphy, S. (1982) 'Self-Help in Middlesborough', *British Tinnitus Association Newsletter,* No. 17, iii–v

Murray, N.E. and Reid, G. (1946) 'Temporary Deafness due to Gunfire', *Journal of Laryngology and Otology, 61,* 92–130

Mycklebust, H.R. (1964) *The Psychology of Deafness,* Grune and Stratton, New York

Myers, E.N. and Bernstein, J.M. (1965) 'Salicylate Ototoxicity', *Archives of Otolaryngology, 82,* 483–93

Mygind, S.H. (1931) 'Buzzing Noise in the Ear', *Acta Otolaryngologica, 15,* 426–32

Nevins, M.A., Lyon, L.J. and Kim, J.M. (1978) 'Multiple Arterial Abnor-malities Presenting as Pulsatile Tinnitus', *Journal of the Medical Society of New Jersey, 75* (6), 467–70

Nodar, R.H. (1978) 'Tinnitus Aurium: An Approach to Classification', *Otolaryngology, 86* (1): ORL–40–46

Northern, J.L. and Zarnoch, J.M. (1979) 'Aural Rehabilitation in Noise Induced Hearing Loss', *Otolaryngologic Clinics of North America, 12,* 693–703

Opitz, H.J. and Von Wedel, H. (1984) 'On the Limited Benefit of Electrical

Stimulation in Tinnitus Suppression', *Archives of Oto-Rhino-Laryngology, 239,* 119

Ouaknine, G.E., Robert, F., Molino-Negro, P. and Hardy, J. (1980) 'Geniculate Neuralgia and Audio-vestibular Disturbances due to Compression of the Intermediate and Eighth Nerves by the Postero-inferior Cerebellar Artery', *Surgical Neurology, 13* (2), 147–50

Pang, L.Q., Pang, M.K. and Takumi, M.M. (1979) 'A New Method of Managing Subjective Tinnitus', *Hawaii Medical Journal, 38* (8), 235–9

Pappas, D.G. (1984) 'Diagnostic Correlations Between Tinnitus and Menière's Disease as Determined by the Computerized Rotary Chair', *Journal of Laryngology and Otology,* Supplement No. 9, Proceedings of the 2nd International Tinnitus Seminar, New York, 10 and 11 June, 1983, pp. 184–7

Parisier, S.C., Chute, P.M., Kramer, S. and Gold, S. (1984) 'Tinnitus in Patients with Chronic Mastoiditis and Cholesteatoma', *Journal of Laryngology and Otology,* Supplement No. 9, Proceedings of the 2nd International Tinnitus Seminar, New York, 10 and 11 June, 1983, pp. 94–7

Parkin, J.L. (1973) 'Tinnitus Evaluation', *American Family Physician, 8* (3), 151–5

Pearson, B.W. and Barber, H.O. (1973) 'Head Injury. Some Otoneurologic Sequelae', *Archives of Otolaryngology, 97* (1), 81–4

Pedersen, U., Bramsen, T. (1984) 'Central Corneal Thickness in Osteogenesis Imperfecta and Otosclerosis', *Oto-Rhino-Laryngology and Opthalmology, 46,* 38–41

Penner, M.J. (1980) 'Two-tone Forward Masking Patterns and Tinnitus, *Journal of Speech and Hearing Research, 23* (4), 779–86

Penner, M.J. (1983) 'The Annoyance of Tinnitus and the Noise Required to Mask It', *Journal of Speech and Hearing Research, 26* (1), 73–6

Penner, M.J., Brauth, S. and Hood, L. (1981) 'The Temporal Course of the Masking of Tinnitus as a Basis for Inferring its Origin', *Journal of Speech and Hearing Research, 24* (2), 257–61

Penner, M.J. (1984) 'Equal-loudness Contours Using Subjective Tinnitus as the Standard', *Journal of Speech and Hearing Research, 27* (2), 274–9

Pilling, M. (1982) 'A Modified Gas-liquid Chromatographic Assay to Monitor Plasma Mexiletine in a Tinnitus Study', *Methods and Findings in Experimental and Clinical Pharmacology, 4,* 243–7

Potthurst, S. (1984) 'The Torment of Tinnitus, *Nursing Mirror, 158* (21), 34–6

Quarry, J.G. (1972) 'Unilateral Objective Tinnitus: A Case and a Cure', *Archives of Otolaryngology, 96* (3), 252–3

Racy, J. and Ward-Racey, E.A. (1980) 'Tinnitus in Imipramine Therapy', *American Journal of Psychiatry, 133* (7), 845–55

Rahko, T. and Hakkinen, V. (1979) 'Carbamazepine in the Treatment of Objective Myoclonus Tinnitus', *Journal of Laryngology and Otology, 93* (2), 123–7

Raskin, M., Johnson, G. and Rondestvedt, J.W. (1973) 'Chronic Anxiety Treated by Feedback-Induced Muscle Relaxation', *Archives of General Psychiatry, 28,* 263–7

Reddel, R.R., Kefford, R.F., Grant, J.M., Coates, A.S., Fox, R.M. and

Tattersall, M.H. (1982) 'Ototoxicity in Patients Receiving Cisplatin: Importance of Dose and Method of Drug Administration', *Cancer Treatment Reports, 66* (1), 19–23

Reich, G. and Johnson, R.M. (1984) 'Personality Characteristics of Tinnitus Patients', *Journal of Laryngology and Otology,* Supplement No. 9, Proceedings of the 2nd International Tinnitus Seminar, New York, 10 and 11 June, 1983, pp. 228–32

Reid, G. (1948) 'Permanent Deafness due to Gunfire', *Journal of Laryngology and Otology, 62,* 76–87

Riedner, E.D. and Young, R.J. (1982) 'Experience with Tinnitus Therapy', *Hearing Instruments, 33,* 28

Robinson, W. (1983) 'New Treatment for Tinnitus', *New Age, 22,* 34–5

Rock, E.H. (1984) 'Forceful Eyelid Closure Syndrome', *Journal of Laryngology and Otology,* Supplement No. 9, Proceedings of the 2nd International Tinnitus Seminar, New York, 10 and 11 June, 1983, pp. 165–9

Roeser, R.J. and Price, D.R. (1980) 'Clinical Experience with Tinnitus Maskers', *Ear and Hearing, 1* (2), 63–8

Ronis, M.L. (1981) 'Menière's Disease and Tinnitus', *Journal of Laryngology and Otology,* Supplement No. 4, 151–2

Ronis, M.L. (1984) 'Inflammatory Ear Disease and Tinnitus', *Journal of Laryngology and Otology,* Supplement No. 9, Proceedings of the 2nd International Tinnitus Seminar, New York, 10 and 11 June, 1983, pp. 203–4

Rose, D.E. (1980) 'Tinnitus Maskers: a Follow-up', *Ear and Hearing, 1* (2), 69–70

Rosenberg, M.E. (1982) *Sound and Hearing,* Edward Arnold, London

Rudin, D.O. (1980) 'Glaucoma, ''Auditory Glaucoma'', ''Articular Glaucoma'' and the Third Eye', *Medical Hypotheses, 6* (4), 427–30

Ruggergo, M.A., Kramek, B. and Rich, N.C. (1984) 'Spontaneous Otoacoustic Emissions in a Dog', *Hearing Research, 13* (3), 293–6

Russell, E.J., Huckman, M. and Rosenberg, M. (1983) 'Sudden Onset of Headache, Proptosis, and Roaring Tinnitus in a Hypertensive 60-year-old Woman', *Journal of the American Medical Association, 249* (23), 3223–4

Salmivalli, A. (1967) 'Acoustic Trauma in Regular Army Personnel: Clinical Audiologic Study', *Acta Otolaryngologica,* Supplement No. 222, 1–85

Saltzman, M. and Ernsner, M.S. (1947) 'A Hearing Aid for the Relief of Tinnitus Aurium', *Laryngoscope, 57,* 358–66

Salvi, R.J. and Ahroon, W.A. (1983) 'Tinnitus and Neural Activity', *Journal of Speech and Hearing Research, 26* (4), 629–32

Sasaki, C.T., Babitz, L. and Kauer, J.S. (1981) 'Tinnitus: Development of a Neurophysiologic Correlate', *Laryngoscope, 91* (2), 2018–24

Sasaki, C.T., Kauer, J.S. and Babitz, L. (1980) 'Differential [14C]2-Deoxyglucose Uptake After Deafferentation of the Mammalian Auditory Pathway — a Model for Examining Tinnitus,' *Brain Research, 194* (2), 511–16

Schleuning, A.J., Johnson, R.M. and Vernon, J.A. (1980) 'Evaluation of a Tinnitus Masking Program: a Follow-up Study of 598 Patients', *Ear*

225

and Hearing, 1 (2), 71–4

Scott, B., Lindberg, P., Lyttkens, L. and Melin, L. (1985) 'Psychological Treatment of Tinnitus. An Experimental Group Study', *Scandinavian Audiology, 14* (4), 223–30

Shambaugh, G.E. Jr. (1977) 'Further Experiences with Moderate Dosage Sodium Fluoride for Sensorineural Hearing Loss, Tinnitus and Vertigo Due to Otospongiosis', *Advances in Otorhinolaryngology, 22*, 35–42

Shapiro, J. (1983) 'Tinnitus', *Talk, 108*, 24–25

Sheps, D.S., Conde, C.A., Mayorga-Cortes, A., Mallon, S.M., Sung, R.J., Castellanos, A. and Myerburg, R.J. (1977) 'Primary Ventricular Fibrillation: Some Unusual Features', *Chest, 72* (2), 235–8

Shulman, A. (1981) 'Clinical Classification of Subjective Idiopathic Tinnitus', *Journal of Laryngology and Otology,* Supplement No. 4, 102–6

Shulman, A. (1981) 'Vasodilator-antihistamine Therapy and Tinnitus Control', *Journal of Laryngology and Otology,* Supplement No. 4, 123–9

Shulman, A. (1984) 'Welcome', *Journal of Laryngology and Otology,* Supplement No. 9, Proceedings of the 2nd International Tinnitus Seminar, New York, 10 and 11 June, 1983, pp. 3–5

Shulman, A. (1984) 'Sub-clinical Tinnitus; Non-auditory Tinnitus', *Journal of Laryngology and Otology,* Supplement No. 9, Proceedings of the 2nd International Seminar, New York, 10 and 11 June, 1983, pp. 77–9

Shulman, A. (1984) 'Relationship of Acoustic Stimulation and Tinnitus Suppression by Electrical Stimulation', *Journal of Laryngology and Otology,* Supplement No. 9, Proceedings of the 2nd International Tinnitus Seminar, New York, 10 and 11 June, 1983, pp. 125–7

Shulman, A. (1984) 'External Electrical Stimulation — Tinnitus Suppression-hearing Preliminary Results', *Journal of Laryngology and Otology,* Supplement No. 9, Proceedings of the 2nd International Tinnitus Seminar, New York, 10 and 11 June, 1983, pp. 141–4

Shulman, A. (1984) 'ABR and Tinnitus — An Overview', *Journal of Laryngology and Otology,* Supplement No. 9, Proceedings of the 2nd International Tinnitus Seminar, New York, 10 and 11 June, 1983, pp. 170–7

Shulman, A. (1984) 'Tinnitus Masking', *Journal of Laryngology and Otology,* Supplement No. 9, Proceedings of the 2nd International Tinnitus Seminar, New York, 10 and 11 June, 1983, pp. 249–56

Simmons, F.B. (1966) 'Electrical Stimulation of the Auditory Nerve in Man', *Archives of Otolaryngology, 84* (1), 2–55

Singerman, B., Riedner, E.D. and Folstein, M. (1980) 'Emotional Disturbance in Hearing Clinic Patients', *British Journal of Psychiatry, 137*, 58–62

Slater, R., Jones, D.M., Terry, A.M.P. and Davis, B.R. (1983) 'Tinnitus Survey: Initial Results from the Tinnitus Research Group, Cardiff', *British Tinnitus Association Newsletter,* No. 20, i–v

Snow, J.B. Jr. (1981) 'Tinnitus and Anatomical Correlates of the Auditory System, Peripheral Centre', *Journal of Laryngology and Otology,* Supplement No. 4, 13–17

Snowden, E. (1981) 'Let's Get This Show on the Road', *British Tinnitus*

Association Newsletter, No. 11, vii–viii

Spitzer, J.B., Goldstein, B.A., Salzbrenner, L.G. and Mueller, G. (1983) 'Effect of Tinnitus Masker Noise on Speech Discrimination in Quiet and Two Noise Backgrounds', *Scandinavian Audiology, 12*, 197–200

Stacey, J.S. (1978) 'Latent Tinnitus?' (Letter), *British Journal of Audiology, 12* (2), 61

Stacey, J.S. (1980) 'Apparent Total Control of Severe Bilateral Tinnitus by Masking, using Hearing Aids', *British Journal of Audiology, 14* (2), 59–60

Steckelberg, J.M. and McDonald, T.J. (1984) 'Otologic Involvement in Late Syphillis', *Laryngoscope, 94* (6), 753–7

Stephens, S.D.G. (1984) 'Historical Origins of the Treatment of Tinnitus', *Soundbarrier*, No. 2, Sept., *British Tinnitus Association Newsletter*, No. 26, 16

Stern, J. and Goldberg, M. (1980) 'Jugular Bulb Diverticula in Medical Petrous Bone', *American Journal of Roentgenology, 134* (5), 959–61

Surr, R.K., Montgomery, A.A. and Mueller, H.G. (1985) 'Effect of Amplification on Tinnitus among New Hearing Aid Users', *Ear and Hearing, 6* (2), 71–5

Svihovec D. and Carmen R. (1982) 'Relaxation-biofeedback Treatment for Tinnitus', *Hearing Instruments, 33*, 32

Sweetow, R. (1985) 'Counselling the Patient with Tinnitus', *Archives of Otolaryngology, 111* (5), 283–4

Tange, R.A. and Bernard, J.L. (1981) 'Tinnitus, a 2000 Hz Dip and a Suspension Vessel in a Scala Tympani', *Clinical Otolaryngology, 6*, 300 (Abstract)

Tange, R.A. and Bernard, J.L. (1981) 'A Cochlear Vascular Anomaly in a Patient with Hearing Loss and Tinnitus', *Archives of Otorhino-laryngology, 233* (2), 117–25

Tees, J.G. (1984) 'Exposure to High Frequency Noise' (letter), *New Zealand Medical Journal, 97* (764), 656–7

Terry, A.M.P., Slater, R., Jones, D.M. and Davis, B.R. (1981) 'Tinnitus Research Group Cardiff: Attempts to Produce Relief from Tinnitus by Using Different Masking Sounds', *British Tinnitus Association Newsletter*, No. 24, 2–4

Tewfig, S. (1974) 'Phonocephalography. An Objective Diagnosis of Tinnitus', *Journal of Laryngology and Otology, 88* (9), 869–75

Tewfig, S. (1983) 'Phonocephalography and Pulsatile Tinnitus in a Surface Cerebral Angioma', *Journal of Laryngology and Otology, 97* (10), 959–62

Thalmann, R. (1975) 'Biochemical Studies of the Auditory System', *Nervous System, 3*, 31–44

Thomsen, J. and Terkildsen, K. (1975) 'Audiological Findings in 125 Cases of Acoustic Neuromas', *Acta Otolaryngologica, 80*, 353–61

Tonndorf, J. (1977) 'A Common Genesis of Hearing Loss, Tinnitus, and Recruitment in a Number of Acute Cochlear Lesions', *Transactions of American Academy of Ophthalmology and Otolaryngology, 84* (2), 475–6

Tonndorf, J. (1980) 'Acute Cochlear Disorders: the Combination of Hearing Loss, Recruitment, Poor Speech Discrimination, and Tinnitus',

227

Annals of Otology Rhinology and Laryngology, 89 (4 Pt. 1), 353–8

Tonndorf, J. (1981) 'Tinnitus and Physiological Correlates of the Cochlea-vestibular System: Peripheral: Central', *Journal of Laryngology and Otology,* Supplement No. 4, 18–20

Tonndorf, J. (1981) 'General Comments', *Journal of Laryngology and Otology,* Supplement No. 4, 97–8

Tonndorf, J. (1981) 'Stereociliar Dysfunction, a Cause of Sensory Hearing Loss, Recruitment, Poor Speech Discrimination and Tinnitus', *Acta Otolaryngologica, 91* (5/6), 469–79

Tonndorf, J. (1984) 'Auditory Coding Mechanisms', *Journal of Laryngology and Otology,* Supplement No. 9, Proceedings of the 2nd International Tinnitus Seminar, New York, 10 and 11 June, 1983, pp. 128–31

Tonndorf, J. and Kurman, B. (1984) 'A New High-frequency Audiometer', *Journal of Laryngology and Otology,* Supplement No. 9, Proceedings of the 2nd International Tinnitus Seminar, New York, 10 and 11 June, 1983, pp. 101–5

Tyler, R.S. and Baker, L.J. (1983) 'Difficulties Experienced by Tinnitus Sufferers', *Journal of Speech and Hearing Disorders, 48,* 150–4

Tyler, R.S. and Conrad-Armes, D. (1983) 'Tinnitus Pitch: A Comparison of Three Measurement Methods', *British Journal of Audiology, 17,* 101–7

Tyler, R.S., Coles, R.A.A. and Haggard, M.P. (1979) 'Tinnitus Research and Treatment: The Role of the Institute of Hearing Research', *British Tinnitus Association Newsletter,* No. 3, i–v

Vernon, J. and Fenwick, J. (1984) 'Identification of Tinnitus: A Plea for Standardization', *The Journal of Laryngology and Otology,* Supplement No. 9, Proceedings of the 2nd International Tinnitus Seminar, New York, 10 and 11 June, 1983, pp. 45–53

Vernon, J. and Fenwick, J. (1984) 'Tinnitus "Loudness" as Indicated by Masking Levels with Environmental Sounds', *Journal of Laryngology and Otology,* Supplement No. 9, Proceedings of the 2nd International Tinnitus Seminar, New York, 10 and 11 June, 1983, pp. 59–63

Vernon, J. and Schleuning, A. (1978) 'Tinnitus: A New Management', *Laryngoscope, 88* (3), 413–9

Vernon, J. *et al.* (1983) 'A Search for Possible Physiological Correlates of Subjective Tinnitus', in R.R. Fay and G. Gouvrevitch (eds.), *Hearing and Other Senses,* Amohora Press, Groton, Connecticut, pp. 385–99

Vernon, J., Schleuning, A., Odell, L. and Hughes, F. (1977) 'A Tinnitus Clinic', *Ear, Nose and Throat Journal, 56* (4), 181–9

Volta, A. (1800) 'On the Electricity Excited by Mere Contact of the Conducting Substances of Difference Kinds', *Transactions of the Royal Society, Philosophy, 90,* 403–31

Walford, R.E. (1980) 'Acoustical Techniques for Diagnosing Low-frequency Tinnitus in Noise Complainants Known as Hummers', *Proceedings of the Institute of Acoustics, 3* (9), 173–86

Walford, R.E. (1982) *Hums and Hummers: A Bibliography of References to Low-frequency Tinnitus, Vascular and Dental Processes, Muscle Tremor, the Microwave Auditory Effect and Low-frequency Sound and Hearing,* Institute of Laryngology, London

Walsh, W.M. and Gerley, P.P. (1985) 'Thermal Biofeedback and the Treatment of Tinnitus', *Laryngology*, 95 (8), 987–9

Ward, P.H. and Honrubia, V. (1969) 'The Effects of Local Anaesthetics on the Cochlea of the Guinea Pig', *Laryngoscope*, 79, 1605–17

Ward, P.H., Babin, R., Calcaterra, T.C. and Konrad, H.R. (1975) 'Operative Treatment of Surgical Lesions with Objective Tinnitus', *Annals of Otology, Rhinology and Laryngology*, 84 (4 Pt. 1), 473–82

Watanabe, I., Kumagami, H. and Tsuda, Y. (1974) 'Tinnitus due to Abnormal Contraction of Stapedial Muscle. An Abnormal Phenomenon in the Course of Facial Nerve Paralysis and its Audiological Significance', *ORL*, 36 (4), 217–26

Von Wedel, H. and Opitz, H.L. (1984) 'Long-term Therapy of Tinnitus with Hearing-aids and Tinnitus-maskers: A Report on Three Years Experience', *Archives of Oto-Rhino-Laryngology*, 239, 119 (Summary)

Wegel, R.L. (1931) 'A Study of Tinnitus', *Archives of Otolaryngology*, 14, 158–65

Weiss, A.D. and Weiss, E.R. (1984) 'Acoustic Trauma: Tinnitus and Vertigo', *Journal of Larnyngology and Otology*, Supplement No. 9, Proceedings of the 2nd International Tinnitus Seminar, New York, 10 and 11 June, 1983. pp. 82–3

Weiss, J.A. (1946) 'Deafness Due to Noises in Warfare', *Naval Medical Bulletin*, 46, 381–6

Whittaker, C.K. (1983) 'Intriguing Change in Tinnitus with Eye Movement', *American Journal of Otology*, 4 (3), 273

Willey, P. (1980) 'A New Outlet', *British Tinnitus Association Newsletter*, No. 5, vii–viii

Wilson, J.P. (1980) 'Recording of the Kemp Echo and Tinnitus from the Ear Canal Without Averaging (Proceedings)', *Journal of Physiology*, 298, 8P–9P

Wilson, J.P. (1984) 'Otoacoustic Emissions and Hearing Mechanisms', *Revue du Laryngologie Otologie Rhinologie*, 105 (2), 179–91

Wood, S. (1982) 'Maskers and Tinnitus Patients', *British Tinnitus Association Newsletter, No. 17*, i–iii

Yamamoto, E., Nishimura, H. and Iwanaga, M. (1985) 'Tinnitus and/or Hearing Loss Elicited by Facial Mimetic Movement', *Laryngoscope*, 95 (8), 966–70

Yanick, P. (1981) 'Tinnitus: A Holistic Approach', *Hearing Instruments*, 32 (7), 12–15, 39

Yanick, P. (1982) 'New Hope for Hearing and Tinnitus Problems: Nutrition and Biochemistry', *Hearing Instruments*, 33, 34

Ylikoski, J., Palva, T. and Virtanen, I. (1977) 'The Morphology of the Vestibular Nerve in a Patient with Normal Vestibular Function and in Patients with Menière's Disease', *Archives of Oto-Rhino-Laryngology*, 215 (1), 45–54

Yoo, T.J., Shea, J.J., Per Lee, J., Shulman, A., Yazawa, Y., Floyd, R., Kuo, C.Y., McCabe, B. and Gardner, G. (1984) 'Autoimmune Inner Ear Disease: A Treatment Update', *Journal of Laryngology and Otology*, Supplement No. 9, Proceedings of the 2nd International Tinnitus Seminar, New York, 10 and 11 June, 1983, pp. 220–7

Yoo, T.J., Tomoda, K., Yazawa, Y., Floyd, R., Stuart, J.M., Cremer, M.,

Ishibe, T., Kang, A.H. and Townes, A.S. (1984) 'Autoimmune Ear Disease: Animal Models Update a Possible Tinnitus Model?', *Journal of Laryngology and Otology,* Supplement No. 9, Proceedings of the 2nd International Tinnitus Seminar, New York, 10 and 11 June, 1983, pp. 205–19

Zelig, S., Deutsch, E. and Eilon, A. (1984) 'Waardenburg Syndrome with Associated Multiple Anomalies', *Journal for Oto-Rhino-Laryngology and its Related Specialities, 46,* 34–7

Glossary of technical terms

Absolute threshold
This usually refers to the lowest intensity at which a pure tone can be detected. The tone would be usually presented in a sound-proof room.

Amplitude
The peak amplitude of a sine wave is the largest value of sound pressure (in air) or the electrical voltage (in sine wave generator). The value at any particular instant is known as instantaneous amplitude.

Audiogram
This is a graph of the absolute threshold plotted against a pure tone frequency. The frequencies used commonly are 125 Hz, 250 Hz, 500 Hz, 1 kHz, 2 kHz, 4 kHz and 8 kHz. For clinical purposes the plot is shown as a hearing loss in dB (difference between average hearing threshold and individual threshold) against frequency.

Bandwidth
Often quoted in terms of octaves. This is the difference between the lowest and highest frequency limits of a noise band where there is energy at all frequencies between these two limits. It can also refer to the width of a filter where the upper and lower frequency limits are defined as the points at which the response is at half-power (or equivalently fallen by 3 dB).

Basilar membrane
A membrane inside the cochlea (inner ear) that is set into vibration by the action of sound-waves on the ear drum and ossicles. Movement of this membrane leads to the production of neural impulses in the auditory pathway.

Beats
When two tones of slightly different frequencies and similar amplitudes are presented they can be perceived as one note, which is fluctuating in amplitude. The change in amplitude is slow when the two frequencies are close and becomes faster as the frequency difference is increased. The rate of change is equal to the frequency difference between the two tones.

Binaural
The use of two ears in a listening task.

Cholesteatoma
A tumour of the membrane of the middle ear.

Cogan's syndrome
A non-syphilitic disease of young adults of rapid onset, which is accompanied by tinnitus, vertigo and deafness.

Combination tone
A combination tone is a tone that is produced as an extra component when two or more tones are presented. Its presence indicates that the processing of the sound complex by the ear is non-linear, e.g. given two primary tones of frequency f1 and f2 where (f2 > f1) an important combination tone is generated by the auditory system at frequency 2f1 − f2. This occurs even at low intensity levels of the presented tones.

Concha (latin word meaning shell)
This refers to the flap at the entrance to the ear canal.

Conductive hearing loss
Deafness resulting from damage or disease of the outer or middle ear.

Dichotic
Presentation of two different sound stimuli to the two ears.

Diotic
Presentation of sound to both ears.

Diplacusis
The condition where the perception of one sound differs between the two ears, e.g. the same tone produces two different pitches in the two ears.

Distortion tone
Distortion products can arise if high-intensity tones are presented to the ear. They are 'extra' to the stimulus and indicate a non-linear transfer function at the upper end of the dynamic range of the ear.

Decibel (dB)

A logarithmic measure of the ratio of one power against a reference power. A convenient working measure suited to the large dynamic range of the ear.

Filter

This is a device for accepting some frequencies and rejecting others. The range of frequencies accepted by the filter is called the passband or bandwidth.

Fundamental frequency

The fundamental frequency of a complex periodic sound corresponds to the period (repetition time) of that sound. A square wave of 100 Hz is made up of a fundamental sinusoidal component at 100 Hz (the fundamental frequency) plus all the odd harmonics of diminishing amplitude.

Hearing level (dB HL)

This is the threshold of hearing for a pure tone at a specified frequency relative to the normal hearing standard. It is used clinically to specify hearing loss.

Hertz (hz)

A unit of frequency equivalent to cycles per second.

Intensity

This is the sound power transmitted through unit area, usually expressed in Watts/cm^2

Linear

In a linear system an increase in input gives rise to a proportional rise in output. This is known as the principle of homogeneity. Also the response to two different input components is the same as adding the response to each input component when presented alone (principle of superposition). For sound systems a linear system will not introduce any 'extra' frequency components other than those present in the input.

Loudness

This is the psychological correlate of intensity. A change of 10 dB is usually perceived as a doubling of loudness.

Loudness level
The loudness level of a sound is quoted in phons, which is the sound pressure level in dB (dB SPL) of a 1 kHz tone which is judged to be equal in loudness to the sound.

Masking
This refers to the ability of one sound to affect the audibility of another sound. Usually the greater the intensity of a sound the greater will be the masking of other sounds. Low-frequency sounds have a greater masking effect on high-frequency sounds than vice versa. This is often referred to by the phrase 'upward spread of masking'.

Menière's Disease
A condition of the inner ear giving rise to symptoms of deafness, tinnitus and vertigo.

Monoaural
A situation where only one ear is involved.

Neuroma
A tumour composed of nerve cells and nerve fibres.

Noise
Usually any unwanted sound, but the term noise-band refers to a non-periodic sound consisting of random fluctuations.

Nystagmus
A reflex scanning movement of the eyes to keep objects in view. In certain conditions when the balance organ of the middle ear is impaired, nystagmus occurs when normally the eyes would be still. This produces vertigo and may lead to nausea.

Octave
A frequency ratio of 2 to 1. Middle 'C' on the piano is 256 Hz. The note an octave above this is also a 'C' but of frequency 512 Hz. A fractional octave is defined by $f1/f2 = 2^n$ where n is a fraction (e.g. 1/3) and $f1 > f2$.

Otitis media
A general term covering a variety of middle ear infections that cause the mucous membrane lining the middle ear to become inflamed and

secrete an excess of fluid, which may sometimes rupture the ear drum.

Periodic sound
This is a sound that is regularly repeating itself exactly in time, e.g. a sine wave where the period = 1/frequency.

Phase
A measure of the stage of a periodic sound. That is, the lead or lag in degrees or radians relative to a fixed point in time or another periodic sound. When two sine waves are added that are of the same frequency and amplitude but which differ in phase by 180 degrees they will cancel each other exactly and no sound will be heard.

Phon
The unit of loudness (see loudness level).

Pitch
The psychological correlate of frequency.

Presbyacusis
A term for the general loss of sensitivity of hearing with age. In general the loss is greatest at the high frequencies.

Recruitment
Loudness recruitment refers to the phenomenom in which the growth of loudness with sound intensity is greater than normal. This usually occurs in a region of hearing loss.

Residual inhibition
This refers to the state where tinnitus loudness is markedly reduced following a period where the tinnitus was masked.

Resonance
Most objects or systems that are capable of vibrating have a natural resonant frequency. This is the frequency at which external vibrations have their maximum effect on the amplitude of vibration. An opera singer can cause a wine glass to break if she sings a note that is close to the resonant frequency of the glass.

Sensation level (SL)
Sensation level is the level in dB of a sound above the audible

threshold. Thus in a region of hearing loss an intense tone may only be a few dB SL.

Sensorineural hearing loss
Hearing loss caused by damage, disease or abnormalities of the sensory (cochlear/inner ear) and/or neural elements of the auditory system.

Sine wave
A wave that varies in the manner of simple harmonic motion. A pure tone.

Sound pressure level
The root-mean-square pressure of a sound expressed in decibels using a reference pressure of 2×10^{-5} Newton/square metre.

Spontaneous activity
The random firing of a neural unit that occurs in the absence of any external stimulus.

Threshold shift
A change in the audibility threshold. This can be temporary or pemanent. The presentation of an intense sound for several minutes will usually cause a temporary threshold shift (TTS). Long-term exposure to intense sound may cause a permanent threshold shift (PTS).

Timbre
The same note produced by difference instruments can be distinguished by its 'timbre', which is derived from the characteristic pattern of the harmonics in amplitude and phase.

Tinnitus masked audiogram
A plot of tone frequency against the tone intensity in dB hearing level required to mask the tinnitus. Such a plot can be useful in categorising the tinnitus.

Tinnitus
A noise that is internally generated by the ear or surrounding tissues and which is perceived by the sufferer.

Waveform
The curve traced by the change of amplitude with time of a sound. A pure tone has a regular periodic waveform.

White noise
Noise that is random statistically and has equal energy at all frequencies (at least over the normal hearing range).

USEFUL ADDRESSES

The British Tinnitus Association (BTA) and the American Tinnitus Association (ATA) have up-to-date lists of local self help groups, of masker manufacturers, and of medical specialists with a stated interest in Tinnitus. They can be contacted at the addresses below:

The Information Officer,
The British Tinnitus Association,
c/o RNID,
105 Gower Street,
London
WC1E 6AH
U.K.

The Information Officer,
The American Tinnitus Association,
P.O. Box 5,
Portland,
Oregon 97207,
U.S.A.

Index